The Muscle Testing Handbook

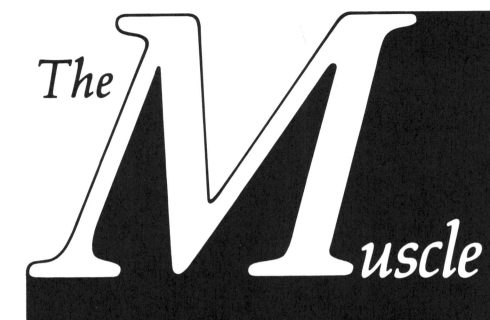

The **M** *uscle*

Virginia Pact, M.D.
Associate in Medicine, Division of Neurology, Duke University Medical Center, Durham, North Carolina

Marcia Sirotkin-Roses, M.A., L.P.T.
Research Associate, Division of Neurology, and Adjunct Assistant Professor, Department of Physical Therapy, Duke University Medical Center, Durham, North Carolina

Joseph Beatus, M.A., L.P.T.
Lecturer, Department of Physical Therapy, University of Maryland, Eastern Shore, Princess Anne, Maryland

Testing Handbook

Forewords by
Sir John Walton, T.D., M.D., D.Sc., F.R.C.P.
Warden, Green College, Oxford; Former Professor of Neurology, University of Newcastle upon Tyne

Allen D. Roses, M.D.
Professor and Chief, Division of Neurology, Duke University Medical Center, Durham, North Carolina

Little, Brown and Company
Boston/Toronto

Library of Congress Catalog Card No. 83-82943

ISBN 0-316-68768-5

Printed in the United States of America

HAL

Contents

Foreword I

I have greatly enjoyed reading this volume and studying the admirable illustrations. In an age of increasing medical technology when diagnosis and differential diagnosis of many diseases, not least those of the neuromuscular system, has proved to be increasingly dependent upon modern sophisticated techniques of investigation involving complex and often expensive biochemical, electrophysiologic, and histologic studies, every doctor, nurse, and physiotherapist with an interest in those diseases that affect skeletal muscle does well to remember that clinical examination of the neuromuscular system, combined with the clinical history, invariably takes one well along the road to accurate diagnosis. Undue reliance upon sophisticated diagnostic tests can often mislead, just as undue reliance upon clinical examination without the availability of complementary diagnostic methods may similarly be dangerous.

Every doctor with experience in examining patients with neuromuscular problems comes increasingly to recognize that specific patterns of muscular wasting and weakness occur in various disease processes, whether these be lesions of isolated peripheral nerves, of multiple peripheral nerves (e.g., polyneuropathy), of the neuromuscular junction (e.g., myasthenia gravis) or of the muscles themselves (e.g., the many varieties of myopathy). Similarly, specific patterns of muscular involvement occur in those diseases that affect specifically the anterior horn cells (e.g., spinal muscular atrophy and amyotrophic lateral sclerosis). Clinical differential diagnosis then is often based upon pattern recognition combined with careful analysis of the patient's personal history and family history. But if this technique is to be effective, then methods of quantitative assessment of muscle power must be applied. This technique of manual muscle testing is a specialized skill, acquired by practice and experience. It behooves any doctor working in this field to develop a technique of his own. This volume describes and illustrates methods of proven value. It will, I am sure, be of value to all interested in this particular field.

Sir John Walton

Foreword II

Sometimes in clinical medicine we miss the obvious because of our familiarity with an old, seemingly reliable way of approaching a problem. Many new advances in the clinical neurosciences have had an impact on our practice, including computerized axial tomography, nuclear magnetic resonance, new biochemical assays, and recombinant DNA techniques. It may, therefore, appear presumptuous to call attention to a new way of examining patients.

In fact, manual muscle testing is not new at all. These techniques date from the poliomyelitis epidemics and have been practiced by physical therapists for many years. The "discovery" of these methods of physical diagnosis came late in my training, well after my residency. Working side by side with one of the co-authors of this manual for 13 years, it became quite clear that the muscle testing that I had learned, designed to identify peripheral nerve injuries, was not precise enough to detect weakness in different muscles innervated by the same nerve or root distribution. The reproducibility of results was suspect, especially when the patient was seen by multiple examiners. This handbook germinated from the need for a vehicle to teach medical students, residents, and other physicians the techniques of manual muscle testing.

Manual muscle testing does not replace other types of examinations. However, if only one method of examination is to be used routinely to record definite slow progression of weakness, our experience emphasizes the manual muscle test. It takes time to learn but has discriminating value in differentiating subtle variations in the presentation of genetic and acquired neuromuscular disease. Manual muscle testing provides a useful, longitudinal measure of increased or decreased strength in chronic diseases. It offers a standardized way of examining relatives of affected patients in pedigrees of genetic or neuromuscular diseases. The techniques are not necessarily more useful when a definite peripheral nerve injury has occurred, and they should be used with care when upper motor neuron signs and spasticity are present.

The techniques of manual muscle testing are extremely valuable as an adjunct to functional testing in following the progression of muscular dystrophies, in discriminating minimal disease expression, in differential diagnosis, and in evaluating response to treatments. In an age of laboratory and radiologic preeminence, manual muscle testing satisfies that part of me that wants to increase the precision of differential diagnosis by history and physical examination.

Allen D. Roses, M.D.

Preface

The Muscle Testing Handbook is intended to be used at the bedside or in the examining room as an easy reference and helpful guide to the techniques of manual muscle testing. There are several fine textbooks available for a more in-depth view [6, 9]. It is the aim of this book to present a method of manual muscle testing useful beyond testing for peripheral nerve injuries [11].

Muscle testing is a skill that can only be acquired with practice. We have provided some fundamental principles and methods in the first section and have illustrated the techniques with photographs of individual muscles in their testing positions. The sequence of muscles tested is designed to speed the examination and to avoid undue patient fatigue (see the Appendix, "Order of the Examination and Alternate Positions").

Young children between the ages of 2 and 5 years often do not have the patience or coordination to participate in muscle testing. Therefore, we have included a section on how to assess functional muscle strength in children through positions and games that the examiner can use with the child. Gross motor skills can be assessed in a child younger than 2 years by using the Denver Developmental Scale [7].

The shoulder and scapula are particularly complex anatomic structures. Some basic principles of kinesiology are illustrated as a background to muscle testing this area. Also discussed in more detail are the thumb and the facial muscles, two often-neglected areas of testing.

To further assist the examiner, we have included charts of the plexuses, major nerves, and dermatomes.

V.P.
M.S.-R.
J.B.

Acknowledgments

The authors wish to thank Dr. Allen Roses, Professor and Chief, Division of Neurology, Duke University Medical Center, for his support, encouragement, and criticisms during the writing of this handbook. We also wish to thank Dr. James Davis, Chief of Neurology, Veteran's Administration Medical Center, Durham, N.C., for his helpful suggestions. We are grateful to the Duke Neurology Residents and to Lisa Trofatter, L.P.T., for their comments and criticisms. Laurie Sawhill, L.P.T., contributed her expertise to the pediatric section, and Wanda Beam, Nancy Holmes, Dee Staples, and Suzanne Parrish contributed their time and skill in typing the manuscript. We also appreciate the cooperation of the Department of Physical Therapy, Duke University Medical Center.

We express our gratitude to Donald Powell, A.M.I., Medical Illustrator, Durham Veteran's Administration Hospital, for his artistry and talent; and to Butch Usery, Senior Medical Photographer, Duke University Medical Center, for the photography.

We are most grateful to Curtis Vouwie, Medical Editor, Little, Brown and Company, for his help and availability during the preparation of the manuscript.

We are indebted to the patients and the families of the Duke Neuromuscular Research Clinic who have cooperated with us and taught us so much through the years.

Finally, our special thanks go to Jeffrey Stajich, P.A.C., and Joanna, Jason, and Michelle, without whose patience and long hours spent in odd positions, this handbook would never have materialized.

V.P.
M.S.-R.
J.B.

The Muscle Testing Handbook

Key to Symbols in Text

Thick arrows (◀■) indicate resistance.
Thin arrows (◀———) indicate muscle belly.
Black and white arrows are used interchangeably, depending on the background of the illustration.

Innervations

   Boldface type indicates major innervation. **C6, C7**, etc.

   Regular type indicates minor innervation. C6, C7, etc.

   Parentheses indicate a variable innervation. (C6), (C7), etc.

Innervations in this text are based on the 35th British Edition of *Gray's Anatomy* (see Bibliography). Innervations may vary depending on the reference used.

The labels for sensory nerves (shown in the drawings by dotted lines) are in italic type. Motor nerves are in regular type.

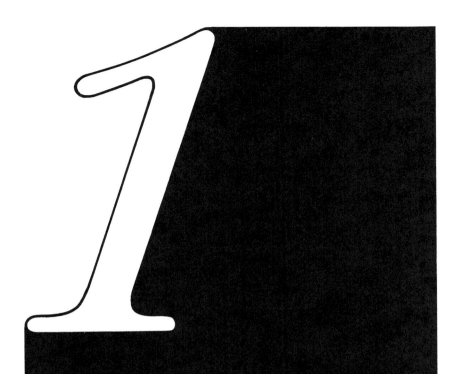

Principles of
the Examination

Fundamentals

In the early 1900s, Dr. Robert W. Lovett, Professor of Orthopedic Surgery at Harvard Medical School, working with patients with poliomyelitis, developed the basics of the manual muscle test [10]. His techniques emphasized the use of gravity and resistance, which are the fundamentals of today's methods of muscle testing.

The examination of the neuromuscular system remains an integral part of physical diagnosis. In the general medical examination, the muscle test often is reduced to a brief functional screening. The specific techniques of the isolated muscle examination have been relegated to the physical therapist [14].

The manual muscle test itself can be used as a screening device. The techniques presented in this manual are simplified and organized. The examiner can test a few specific muscles and expand the evaluation as indicated.

Positioning the Patient

Positioning the patient and the body part are key factors for adequate evaluation. The patient should be comfortably positioned on a firm surface and appropriately dressed to allow visualization of the muscles. Not all patients can be tested using standardized positions. Bedbound patients may be tested in the supine or side-lying position, although this does not allow many muscles to be tested with gravity as a grading factor. In this case, strength grades can only be approximated.

Assessing Range of Motion

Before beginning the muscle test, the examiner should assess the range of motion of the involved joint. The patient should be asked to move the body part actively. While the patient is moving the limb, the quality of the movement should be observed: Is it smooth, rapid, bradykinetic, or ataxic? Is there a tremor? The examiner also should observe the muscle bulk: Is there asymmetry, hypertrophy, or atrophy? Are there fasciculations? If active range of motion is restricted, the following must be considered:

Pain (arthritis, soft-tissue inflammation)
Joint tightness (adhesions, swelling)
Muscle contractures

If there is restriction in the active range of motion, the examiner should evaluate muscle tone while passively moving the body part through its range. Is there spasticity, rigidity, or hypotonia? Passive range of motion may be restricted not only by joint disease but also by tight antagonistic muscles. Muscle strength can be tested and graded within the restricted range of motion but should be noted as such. Some fixed contractures still allow for good muscle strength.

Gravity

Most major muscle groups function to move the body part against gravity. Nevertheless, many clinicians do not consider gravity when testing. For example, the triceps often is tested with the subject's arm flexed at the elbow. The subject is asked to push forward into the examiner's hand while trying to extend the elbow against the examiner's counterforce (Fig. 1-1). We consider this invalid for several reasons:

As the forearm moves forward, it is pulled downward by gravity, which assists in moving the limb.
The triceps starts in a position of maximal stretch. Thus, contractile force is already reduced.
The subject usually pushes the shoulder forward and leans his or her body weight against the examiner's resistive force.

The practice of testing muscles in functional positions is useful only when screening for normal strength. If any weakness is detected, the subject should be placed in the antigravity position and assessed for an accurate grade. If the muscle strength is not sufficient to overcome the force of gravity, the subject should be placed in a gravity-eliminated position (see the appendix, "Order of the Examination and Alternate Positions") [6].

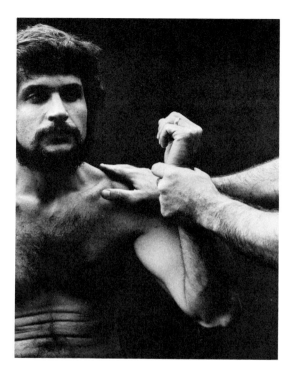

Figure 1-1. Incorrect Position for Testing the Triceps Brachii.

Fixation

To test a distal muscle properly, the proximal limb should be stabilized. If the origin of the muscle is unstable, it will not adequately perform the movement; its contractile pull is at a disadvantage. In the normal subject, a secondary action of many muscles is to help stabilize (fixate) the joint or body part so that the primary movers can function optimally. For example, the wrist extensors stabilize the wrist in neutral, allowing the finger abductors (dorsal interossei and abductor digiti minimi) to function with full strength. If there is a wrist drop (radial nerve palsy), the dorsal interossei cannot be tested in isolation unless the hand and wrist are manually fixated in neutral. The reader should try to abduct his or her fingers both with the wrist in neutral and with the wrist flexed. The limited range of motion and strength of finger abduction in the latter position will be immediately apparent.

In muscle testing, the examiner often needs to manually fixate a proximal part. The muscles of the glenohumeral joint are dependent on the stability of the scapula. If the scapula muscles are weak, the glenohumeral muscles will not function optimally. An example of this interrelationship is shown in Figures 1-2 through 1-4 (see pages 8–9). Sometimes the subject's weight alone provides sufficient stabilization. In testing hip flexion, for instance, the subject's body weight helps stabilize the pelvis in the sitting position.

Grading

The examiner must acquire skill in grading normal subjects of both sexes and all ages [13]. This cannot be overemphasized. Some muscles in normal individuals are surprisingly weak. The middle trapezius in women and the iliopsoas in obese subjects may take very little resistance before "breaking." This may be a normal situation rather than evidence of subtle muscle weakness. This is also true for other muscles in the body, and only experience can differentiate normal strength from mild weakness, taking into account age, sex, and body build.

Many grading systems have been developed, all based on the gravity-resistance techniques introduced by Dr. Lovett [10]. The most frequently used by physicians are the Medical Research Council (MRC) scale [11] and the Kendall scale [9], as numerical symbols are easier to interpret than words (Table 1-1). Half-grades, such as 4+ or 4−, often are used to "fine-grade" muscle strength. These reflect the subjective bias of each experienced examiner based on his or her perception of normal strength for individuals. Muscle-strength testing may vary up to half a grade between examiners but should never vary as much as a whole grade.

Weak muscles fatigue easily and, in a detailed muscle examination, some muscles may grade lower than their true strength if the patient is tiring. Pain, swelling, and cramping in the tested region will interfere with the examination and may inhibit muscle contraction. The examiner should note this in the evaluation.

We feel that the standard muscle testing method presented in this book is applicable to all adults, even those who are superstrong in comparison to the examiner. There are times when there is mild weakness in the muscle of even such an individual. When checking for strength symmetry, the examiner may be unable to discern any difference. In this case, the examiner may need to resort to a more sensitive technique. Mechanical devices, such as the Cybex machine [5],

Table 1-1. *Grading scales*

Definition	Functional description	Grading system		
		MRC	Lovett	Kendall
No movement; no fibers palpable	No movement	0	0	0%
No movement of the part; can palpate minimal contraction	Severe weakness	1	Trace	20%
Movement but not against gravity	Severe weakness	2*	Poor	40%
Full ROM against gravity, but cannot sustain resistance	Moderate weakness	3	Fair	60%
Full ROM against gravity and can take some resistance	Mild weakness	4	Good	80%
Normal strength	Normal	5	Normal	100%

*The muscle should be assessed in a gravity eliminated position if graded less than 3.
MRC = Medical Research Council; ROM = range of motion.

are used to quantitatively evaluate force output. Serial recordings with a dynamometer also can assist in detecting small differences in muscle strength.

Resistance

The examiner may apply either isotonic or isometric resistance. Isotonic resistance is given as the muscle moves through its range. The isometric test is performed at one position in the range of motion, usually where the muscle can produce maximum force. This is known as the *break test* [6]. For accuracy, simplicity, and consistency, we have chosen the isometric technique. A muscle contraction should be smooth when resistance is applied. If there is jerkiness or "giveway," the patient may not be cooperating fully. In this case, the muscle should be checked in a functional position. For example, if the hip abductors appear to be weak, testing for lateral pelvic tilt (Trendelenburg sign) may be useful. If the dorsiflexors of the ankle appear weak, the patient might be asked to walk on his or her heels.

Substitution

If weakness is present, the patient may initiate or try to maintain a position by substituting a stronger muscle for the one being tested. For example, if the biceps brachii is weak, the patient may try to pronate the forearm and use the brachioradialis to flex the elbow.

If too much resistance is applied, even the normal individual may break or deviate from the initial antigravity position. In testing hip flexion, for instance, if too much resistance is applied in a downward direction, the subject may bend forward in an effort to maintain the knee at its set height. The examiner should observe these postural adjustments and reduce the resistance accordingly. Only experience can determine whether the altered posture is due to weakness on the part of the patient or overexuberance on the part of the examiner.

The Shoulder and Scapula

The muscles of the shoulder and scapula are functionally integrated to produce complex movements. The basic kinesiology of these movements must be understood before isolated muscles in this region can be tested. For a more complete discussion of shoulder kinesiology, the reader is referred to several excellent sources [2, 3, 4, 8].

The scapula forms a physiologic joint with the thoracic wall. There are no ligaments to hold the scapula in place; the only joint attachment to the skeleton is the sternoclavicular joint. All other attachments are muscular.

The glenohumeral joint is highly mobile. Its stability depends on its capsular and muscular attachments. Many of these muscles insert on the scapula. Therefore, full range of motion of the glenohumeral joint is dependent on concomitant movement of the scapula. For example, the patient in Figures 1-2 through 1-4 has an unstable scapula which cannot *upwardly rotate* due to weakness of the serratus anterior and the upper and lower trapezius. As a result, she is able to flex the arm forward to only 90 degrees (Fig. 1-3). When the examiner manually fixates the scapula, she is able to elevate her arm to 160 degrees (Fig. 1-4).

8

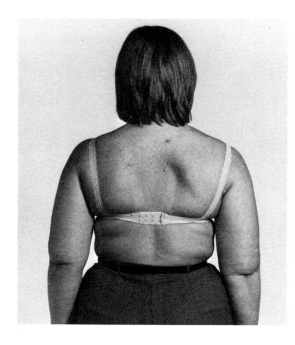

Figure 1-2. Patient
with Unstable Scapula
and Weakness of the
Serratus Anterior.

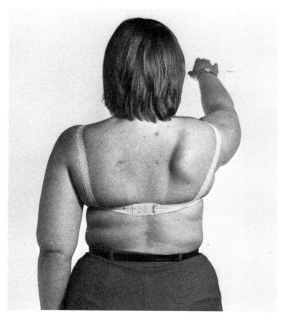

Figure 1-3. Limited
Forward Flexion of the
Arm to 90 Degrees.

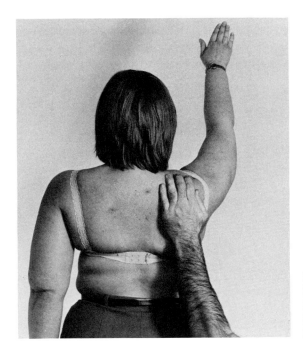

Figure 1-4. With Manual Fixation of the Scapula, Arm Can Be Elevated to 160 Degrees.

With controlled lowering of the arm (as in chopping wood), scapula and glenohumeral joint movements are again interdependent. The scapula must *downwardly rotate* so that its inferior angle is pulled medially (Fig. 1-5).

Other scapular movements include:

Elevation, as in shoulder shrug, performed by the upper trapezius and levator scapulae.

Depression (active), as in pushing down to raise the body up (using crutches or the parallel bars), performed primarily by the lower trapezius and the latissimus dorsi. (Another example, elevation on the hands, is provided in Chapter 8, page 135).

Protraction, performed by the serratus anterior and pectoralis minor (Figure 1-6).

Retraction, performed by the middle trapezius and the rhomboids (Fig. 1-7).

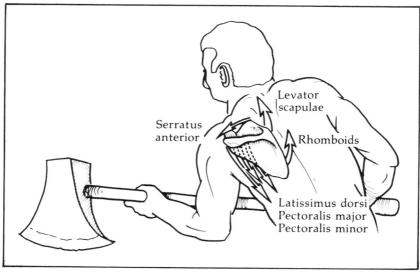

Figure 1-5. Downward Rotation of the Scapula.
(Adapted from Karpandji [8].)

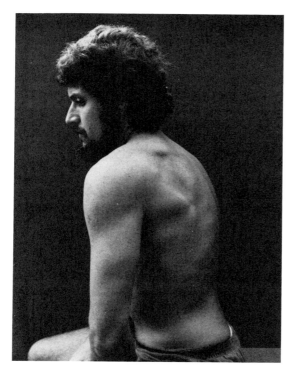

Figure 1-6. Protraction of the Scapula.

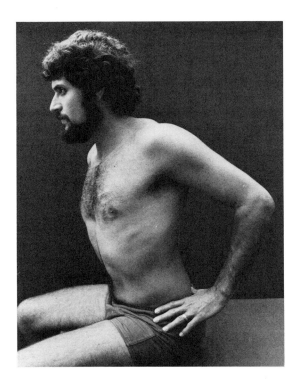

Figure 1-7. Retraction of the Scapula.

There are eight individual directions of movement of the gleno-humeral joint:

Forward flexion, performed primarily by the anterior deltoid, the clavicular head of the pectoralis major, the coracobrachialis, and the long head of the biceps brachii.

Extension, performed primarily by the posterior deltoid (Fig. 1-8).

Abduction, performed primarily by the middle deltoid and the supraspinatus.

Adduction, passive movement, performed by gravity alone, or active movement, performed by the pectoralis major, teres major, and latissimus dorsi (Fig. 1-9).

External (lateral) rotation, performed primarily by the infraspinatus and teres minor.

Internal (medial) rotation, performed primarily by the subscapularis, assisted by the latissimus dorsi, pectoralis major, and teres major (Fig. 1-10).

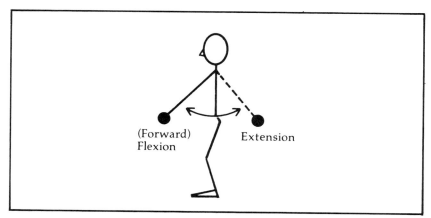

Figure 1-8. Flexion and Extension at the Glenohumeral Joint.

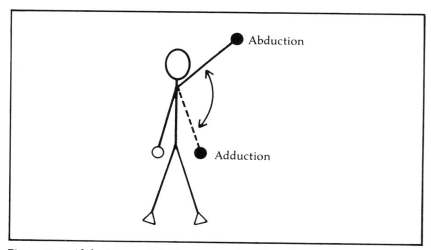

Figure 1-9. Abduction and Adduction at the Glenohumeral Joint.

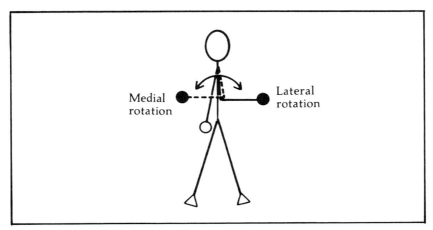

Figure 1-10. Medial and Lateral Rotation at the Glenohumeral Joint.

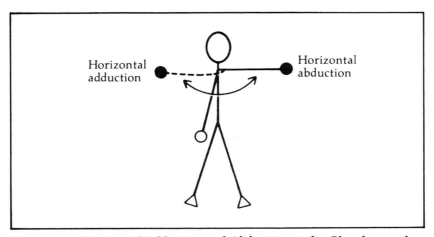

Figure 1-11. Horizontal Adduction and Abduction at the Glenohumeral Joint.

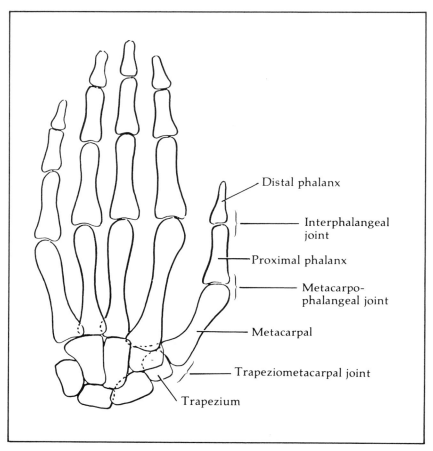

Figure 1-12. Bones and Joints of the Thumb.

Horizontal abduction, performed by the posterior deltoid (Fig. 1-11).
Horizontal adduction, performed by the pectoralis major (sternal head) and the coracobrachialis (Fig. 1-11).

The Thumb

The thumb has a saddle joint which allows for great dexterity and freedom of movement. All primary movements occur at the trapezio-

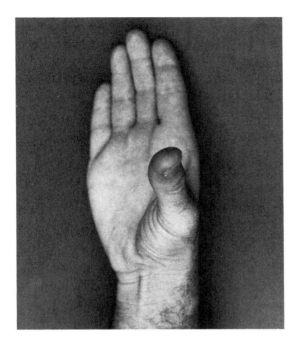

Figure 1-13. Abduction of the Thumb.

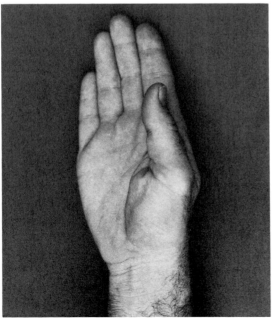

Figure 1-14. Adduction of the Thumb.

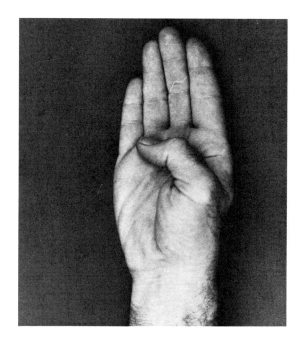

Figure 1-15. Flexion of the Thumb.

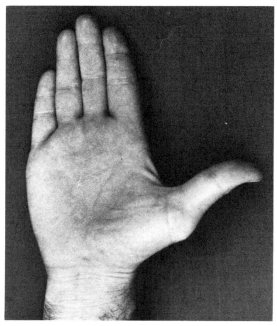

Figure 1-16. Extension of the Thumb.

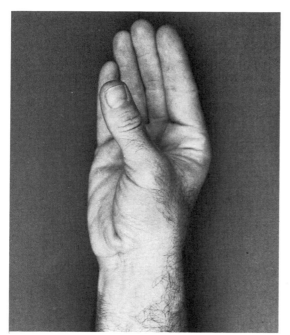

Figure 1-17. Opposition of the Thumb.

metacarpal joint and include *flexion, extension, abduction, adduction,* and *opposition.* These are defined in relation to the supinated outstretched palm. The metacarpophalangeal joint allows for flexion, extension, and some lateral movement away from or toward the plane of the palm (Fig. 1-12).

The extrinsic muscles of the thumb originate in the forearm and are influenced by the position of the wrist. These are the extensor pollicis longus, the extensor pollicis brevis, the abductor pollicis longus, and the flexor pollicis longus.

The intrinsic muscles of the thumb provide stability for the metacarpophalangeal joint and allow the distal muscles to work while the thumb is held in opposition. They are shorter than the extrinsic muscles and originate in the hand itself. They are the opponens pollicis, adductor pollicis, abductor pollicis brevis, flexor pollicis brevis, and one head of the first dorsal interosseus.

The cardinal planes of movement of the thumb are shown in Figures 1-13 through 1-17.

Testing the thumb requires careful palpation, stabilization, and joint positioning. There are *no pure* isolated movements of the thumb. For example, while testing thumb flexion, if resistance applied to the proximal phalanx is increased, the long flexor, which runs deep to the short flexor, will be recruited as well. Similarly, thumb adduction is assisted by the first dorsal interosseous. Opposition is a combined movement of the opponens pollicis and the flexor pollicis brevis. When this movement is resisted, the adductor pollicis and flexor pollicis longus come into play.

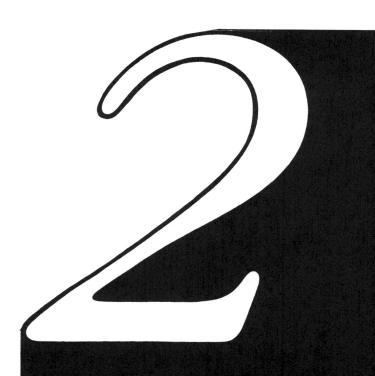

2

Testing in the
Sitting Position

Figure 2-1. Upper Trapezius

Function: *Elevation of the scapula.*

Innervation: *Accessory nerve (cranial nerve XI).*

Comment: *The upper trapezius raises the shoulder up toward the ear. In testing (A), the subject should not push down on the table with his hands. When this muscle is tested unilaterally (B), the subject's head is stabilized by the examiner so that movement is clearly at the shoulder.*

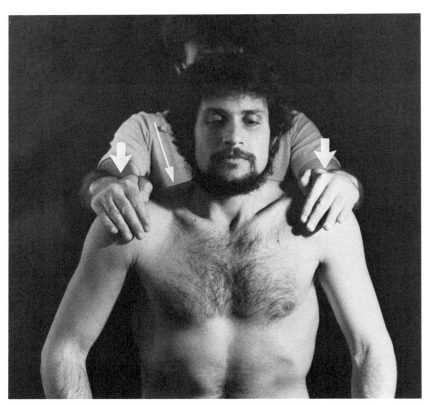

A

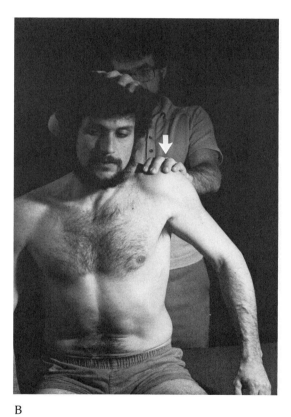

B

22

Figure 2-2. Anterior Deltoid

Function: Forward flexion of the arm.

Innervation: Axillary nerve, **C5**, C6.

Comment: The subject holds the arm midway between flexion and abduction, thus reducing the assistance of the pectoralis major and emphasizing the anterior deltoid fibers. Resistance is applied in a downward and posterior direction.

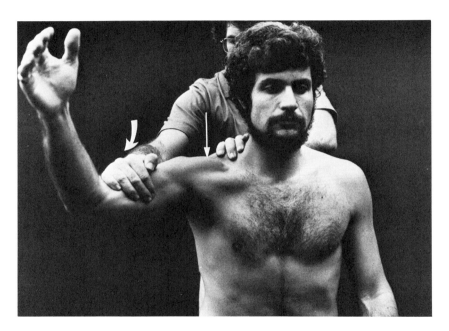

Figure 2-3. Middle Deltoid

Function: *Abduction of the shoulder.*

Innervation: *Axillary nerve,* **C5***, C6.*

Comment: *The middle deltoid is the primary abductor of the arm and is assisted by the supraspinatus. The subject's elbow may be flexed or extended (A). The examiner is stabilizing the scapula (B).*

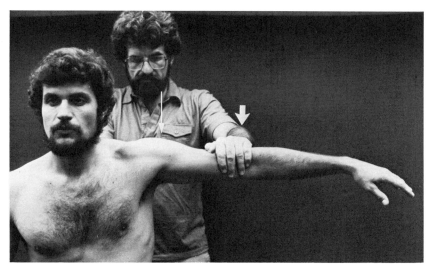

A

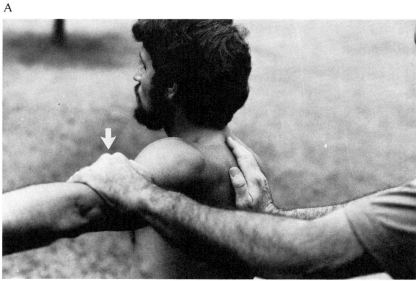

B

Figure 2-4. Supraspinatus

Function: *Assists in shoulder abduction.*

Innervation: *Suprascapular nerve, C4, **C5**, C6.*

Comment: *The supraspinatus cannot be tested in isolation. It is best palpated in the first*
                      15 degrees of abduction, when the trapezius is most relaxed. It also helps to
                      stabilize the head of the humerus into the glenoid cavity. (This patient
                      is able to abduct his arm to 90 degrees with his supraspinatus muscle as his
                      deltoid is completely atrophied.)

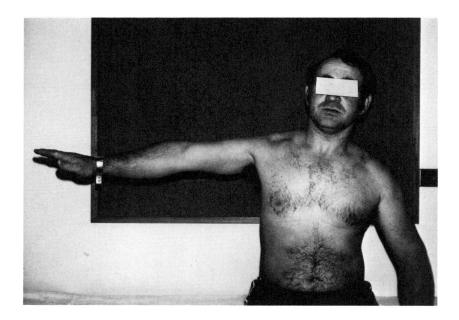

Figure 2-5. Biceps Brachii

Function: Elbow flexion and supination.

Innervation: Musculocutaneous nerve, C5, **C6**.

Comment: The examiner holds the elbow into the trunk for stabilization (A). Resistance is applied gradually at approximately 100 degrees of elbow flexion in a downward direction toward the floor. This muscle should not break for a grade of 5. In this nonstandardized position (B), the examiner does not stabilize the subject. The muscle is at the end of its range and is not performing maximally. Here the examiner pries open the arm by leaning back.

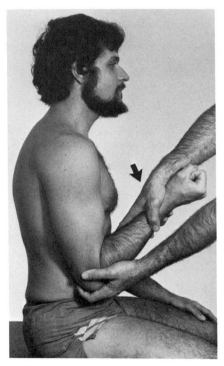

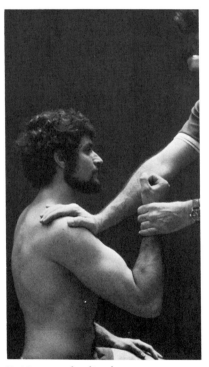

A. Correct   B. Nonstandardized

Figure 2-6. Brachioradialis

Function: *Assists in elbow flexion.*

Innervation: *Radial nerve, C5, **C6**, (C7).*

Comment: *The subject holds his arm midway between supination and pronation. The examiner provides stabilization by holding the elbow into the subject's waist and applies resistance in a downward direction. This muscle does not function in isolation if the biceps brachii is strong.*

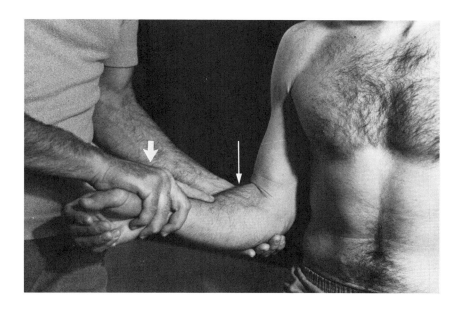

Figure 2-7. Triceps Brachii

Function: *Elbow extension.*

Innervation: *Radial nerve, C6, **C7**, **C8**.*

Comment: *The examiner supports the arm proximal to the elbow (A). The subject straightens his elbow, and the examiner applies resistance distally in a downward direction. The subject keeps his shoulder internally rotated so that the thumb points down. This muscle should not break for a grade of 5. The triceps can also be tested in the prone position (B). The examiner stabilizes the arm under the elbow and applies resistance in a downward direction. (C) Incorrect test of triceps brachii, in which the subject pushes forward into the examiner's hand while trying to extend his elbow against the examiner's counterforce. See also page 3.*

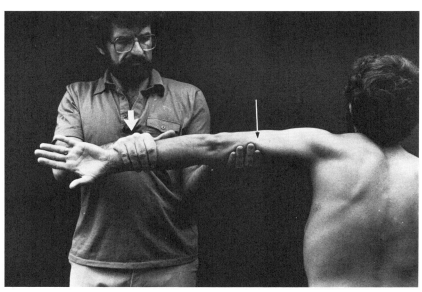

A. Correct

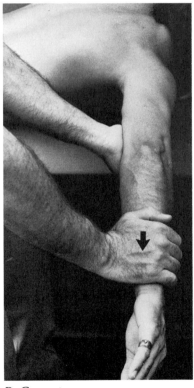

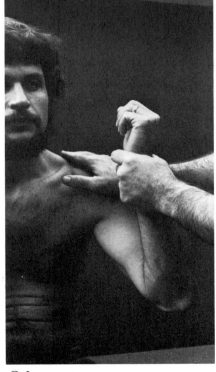

B. Correct

C. Incorrect

Figure 2-8. Supinator

Function: *Supination of the forearm (turning the palm up).*

Innervation: *Radial nerve, C5, **C6**.*

Comment: *The examiner stabilizes the arm at the elbow and applies resistance at the distal forearm in the direction of pronation (A). The supinator is difficult to palpate because it is deep in the forearm. The biceps is a stronger supinator, especially in the position of elbow flexion. (B) Incorrect test of the supinator. Grasping the hand causes the subject to grip firmly, and movement occurs at the wrist, testing the wrist musculature.*

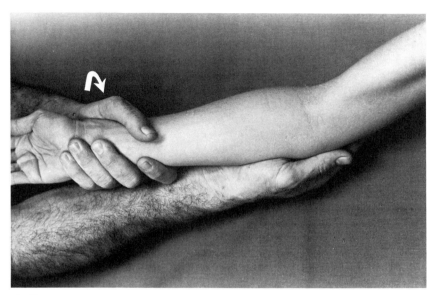

A. Correct

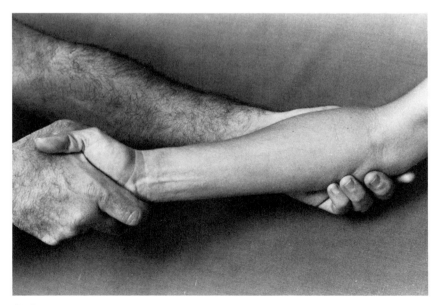

B. Incorrect

Figure 2-9. Pronator Teres

Function: *Pronation of the forearm (turning the palm down).*

Innervation: *Median nerve, C6, **C7**.*

Comment: *The examiner stabilizes the arm at the elbow and applies resistance at the distal forearm in a supinating direction (A). The pronator teres usually is much stronger than the supinator. (B) Incorrect test of this muscle. Grasping the hand causes the subject to grip firmly, and movement occurs at the wrist, testing the wrist musculature.*

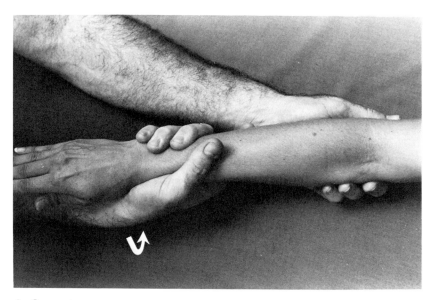

A. Correct

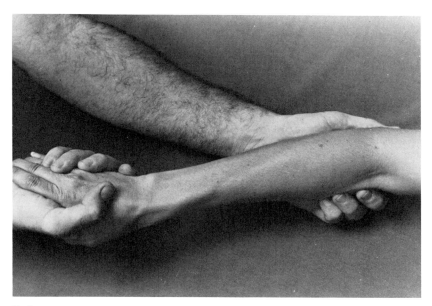

B. Incorrect

Figure 2-10. Wrist Extensors *(extensor carpi radialis longus and brevis, extensor carpi ulnaris)*

Function: Wrist extension.

Innervation: Radial nerve, C6, C7, C8.

Comment: This figure depicts the combined musculature. The examiner stabilizes the forearm. Resistance is applied on the dorsum of the hand on either the radial or the ulnar side. The wrist extensors should not break for a grade of 5. Resistance may be applied with the palm of the examiner's hand.

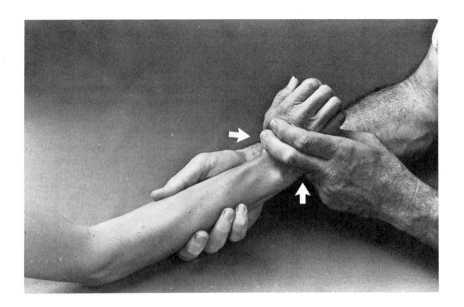

Figure 2-11. Wrist Flexors *(flexor carpi radialis, flexor carpi ulnaris)*

Function:	*Flexion of the wrist.*
Innervation:	*Flexor carpi radialis (A): median nerve, C6, **C7**. Flexor carpi ulnaris (B): ulnar nerve, C7, **C8**.*
Comment:	*Resistance is applied in a radial (A) or ulnar (B) direction. The fingers are maintained in an extended posture as the finger flexors cross the wrist and assist in wrist flexion.*

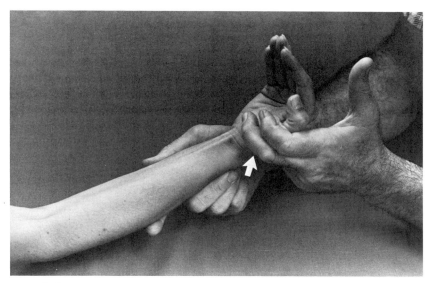

A. Radial

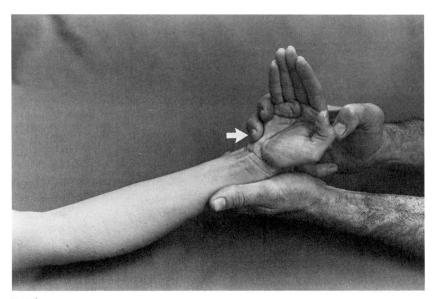

B. Ulnar

Figure 2-12. Finger Extensors *(extensor digitorum, extensor indicis,*
extensor digiti minimi)

Function: *Extension of the fingers.*
Innervation: *Posterior interosseous nerve (from the radial nerve), C7, C8.*
Comment: *The examiner provides stabilization at the wrist to minimize assistance by*
the wrist extensors. Resistance is given distal to the metacarpophalangeal joint.
Fingers can be tested individually.

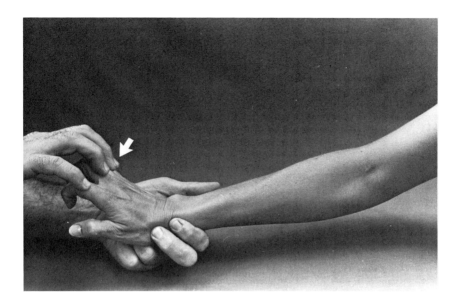

Figure 12-13A. Finger Flexors *(flexor digitorum superficialis)*

Function: Flexion of the fingers at the proximal interphalangeal (PIP) joint.

Innervation: Median nerve, C7, **C8**, T1.

Comment: The examiner is stabilizing three fingers to test each finger individually.
                 Resistance is applied distal to the PIP joint.

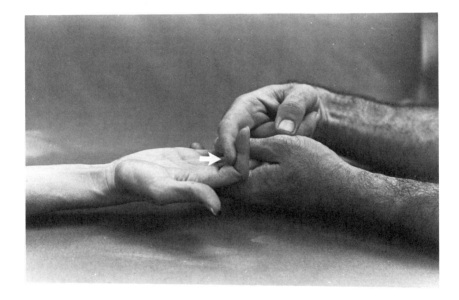

A

Figure 2-13B. Finger Flexors *(flexor digitorum profundus)*

Function: Flexion of the fingers at the distal interphalangeal joint.

Innervation: Digits I and II: Median nerve, **C8**, T1. Digits III and IV: Ulnar nerve, **C8**, T1.

Comment: The examiner provides stabilization at the proximal interphalangeal joint and applies resistance to the distal phalanx. The flexor digitorum profundus takes relatively little resistance.

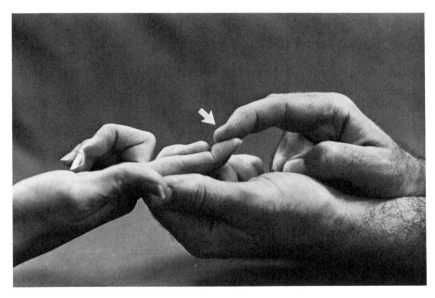

B

Figure 2-13C. Finger Flexors
Functional test of grip strength combining all the finger flexors.

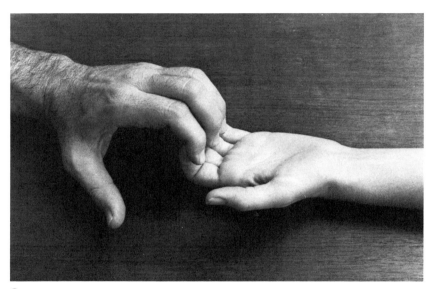

C

Figure 2-14. Dorsal Interossei

Function: *Finger abduction (spreading the fingers apart).*
Innervation: *Ulnar nerve, C8,* **T1***.*
Comment: *The first dorsal interosseous is the strongest of this group in the normal subject. The belly of this muscle is easily seen and palpated. There are four dorsal interossei. Note the abductor digiti minimi abducts the fourth digit.*

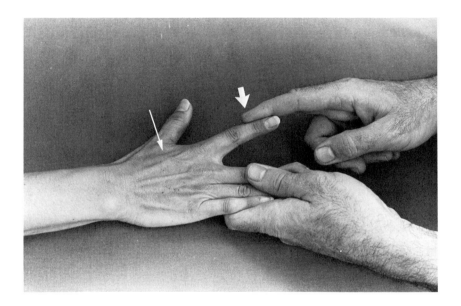

Figure 2-15A. Abductor Digiti Minimi

Function: *Abduction of the fourth digit.*

Innervation: *Ulnar nerve, C8, **T1**.*

Comment: *For the abductor digiti minimi to function maximally, the wrist should remain in the neutral position with the hand flat on the table. With weak wrist extensors, the examiner must stabilize the wrist.*

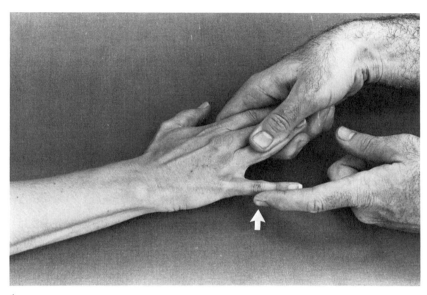

A

Figure 2-15B. First Dorsal Interosseous and Abductor Digiti Minimi
Functional test of two finger abductors simultaneously.

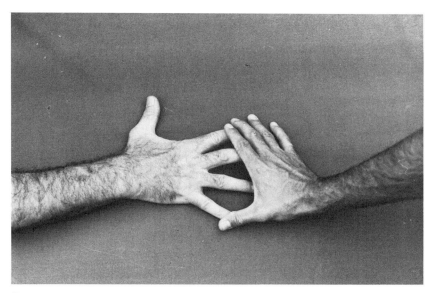

B

Figure 2-16. Palmar Interossei

Function: *Adduction of the fingers (closing the fingers together).*

Innervation: *Ulnar nerve, C8, **T1**.*

Comment: *There are three palmar interossei, none of which inserts on the middle finger. Each one must be tested individually. These muscles work with the lumbricals when flexing the metacarpophalangeal joints.*

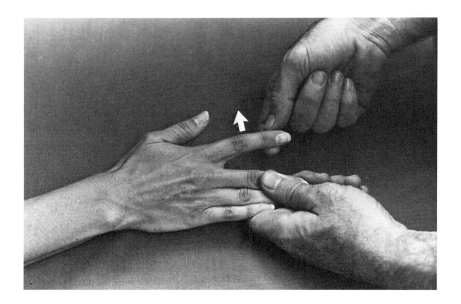

Figure 2-17. Lumbricals

Function: *Flexion of the metacarpophalangeal joint.*

Innervation: *Digits I and II: Median nerve, C8, **T1**. Digits III and IV: Ulnar nerve, C8, **T1**.*

Comment: *There are four lumbricals. The examiner should stabilize the hand at the wrist and ask the subject to flex the fingers to 90 degrees. This group can be tested together.*

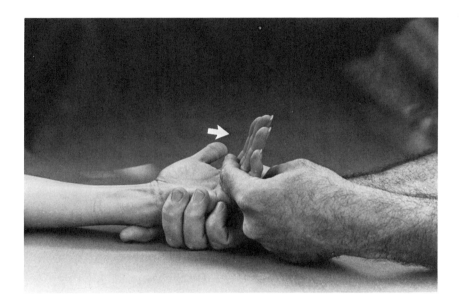

Figure 2-18. Flexor Pollicis Brevis

Function: *Flexion of the proximal phalanx of the thumb.*

Innervation: *Superficial head: Median nerve,* **C8**, *T1. Deep head: Ulnar nerve, C8,* **T1**.

Comment: *The examiner stabilizes the hand. The subject is flexing the proximal phalanx of the thumb. The flexors of the thumb assist in opposition.*

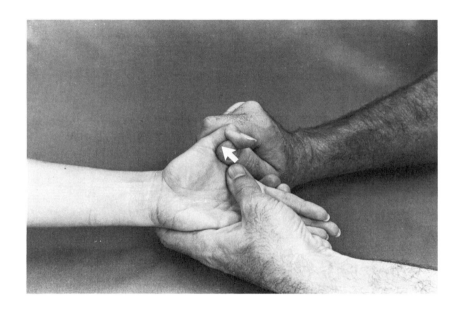

Figure 2-19. Flexor Pollicis Longus

Function: *Flexion of the distal phalanx of the thumb.*

Innervation: *Anterior interosseous branch of the median nerve,* **C8**, *T1.*

Comment: *The examiner stabilizes the proximal joint of the thumb and asks the subject to flex the distal phalanx. The long and short flexors are strong muscles and should hold.*

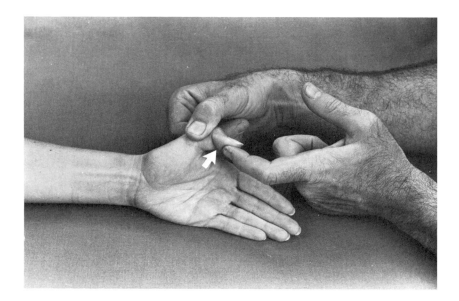

Figure 2-20. Abductor Pollicis Brevis

Function: *Thumb abduction.*

Innervation: *Median nerve,* **C8**, *T1.*

Comment: *The examiner stabilizes the hand to allow movement at the metacarpo-phalangeal joint only. Resistance is applied at the metacarpophalangeal joint in a direction perpendicular to the palm.*

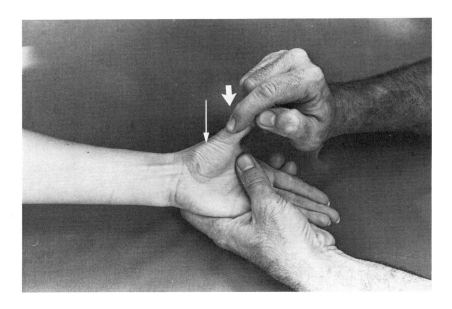

Figure 2-21. Abductor Pollicis Longus

Function: *Abduction of the thumb.*

Innervation: *Posterior interosseous nerve (from the radial nerve), C7, **C8**.*

Comment: *The examiner is stabilizing the wrist to prevent wrist and finger movement.*
                 Resistance is applied proximal to the metacarpophalangeal joint.

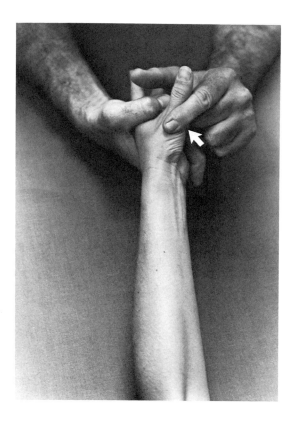

52

Figure 2-22. Extensor Pollicis Brevis

Function: Extension of the thumb (as in hitchhiking).

Innervation: Posterior interosseous nerve (from the radial nerve), C7, **C8**.

Comment: The examiner stabilizes the wrist and hand. Resistance is applied at the proximal phalanx. This tendon runs with the abductor pollicis longus to form the radial border of the anatomic snuffbox.

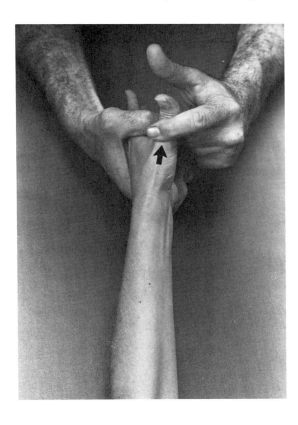

Figure 2-23. Extensor Pollicis Longus

Function: *Extension of the thumb.*

Innervation: *Posterior interosseous nerve (from the radial nerve), C7,* **C8.**

Comment: *The examiner provides stabilization at the wrist and hand and applies resistance to the distal phalanx in the direction of flexion. The tendon forms the ulnar border of the anatomic snuffbox.*

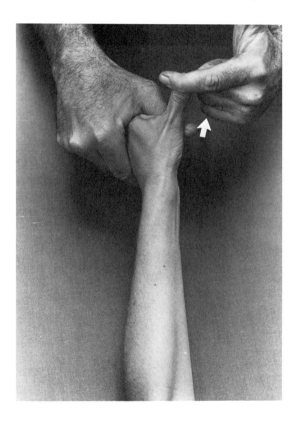

Figure 2-24. Opponens Pollicis

Function: *Bringing the thumb across the palm toward the fourth digit (opposition).*

Innervation: *Median nerve,* **C8**, *T1.*

Comment: *Resistance is given to the muscular part of the thumb, against the metacarpal bone (A). This is a very strong muscle and should not break. (B) Incorrect test of the opponens pollicis. This photograph demonstrates a combined action of the long and short flexors of the thumb and fourth digit, as well as opposition. In this position, the examiner can easily pull his or her finger through the subject's fingers. Thus, this is not a true test for these very strong muscles.*

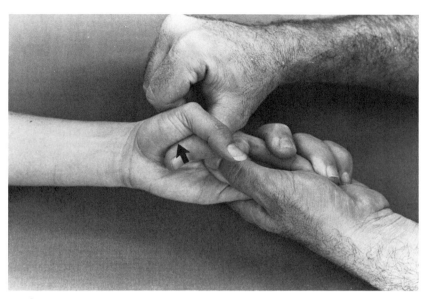

A. Correct

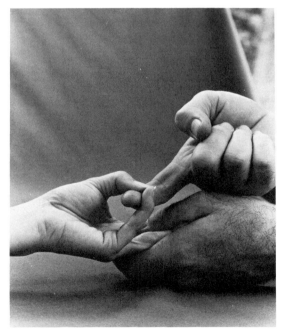

B. Incorrect

Figure 2-25. Adductor Pollicis

Function: *Approximation of the thumb to the palm of the hand.*

Innervation: *Ulnar nerve, C8,* **T1**.

Comment: *The examiner stabilizes the fingers and asks the subject to adduct the thumb from a starting position of abduction (as shown). One may also start with the thumb on the palm (fully adducted) and apply resistance in the direction of abduction. The thumb should not be allowed to flex.*

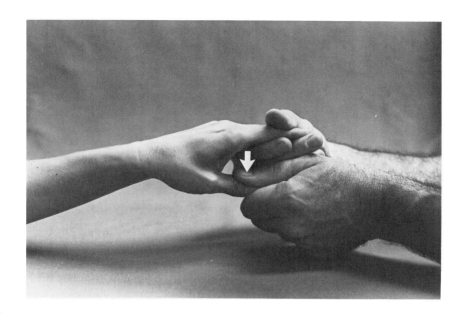

Figure 2-26. Iliopsoas

Function:	*Hip flexion.*
Innervation:	*Femoral nerve, and ventral rami of lumbar nerves, **L1**, **L2**, L3.*
Comment:	*The subject is asked to raise his leg to no more than 45 degrees off the table (A). Hip abduction or rotation should be avoided (to minimize the contribution of the tensor fasciae latae and sartorius). Obese subjects may have difficulty with this position. In some older women, this muscle cannot withstand very strong resistance. (B) Nonstandardized position for testing the iliopsoas. It may be used for bed-bound patients. It is not an antigravity position.*

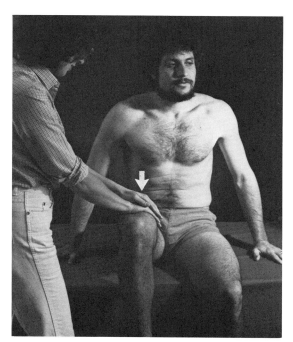

A. Correct

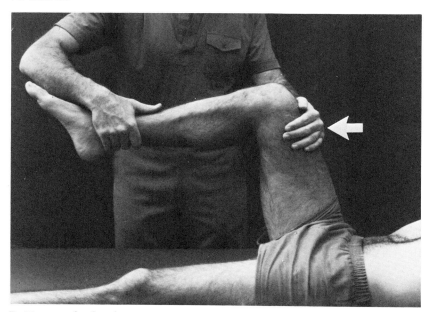

B. Nonstandardized

Figure 2-27. Internal Rotators of the Hip *(gluteus medius, gluteus minimus,*
tensor fasciae latae)

Function: Internal (medial) rotation of the hip.
Innervation: Superior gluteal nerve, L4, L5, S1.
Comment: The subject is asked to hold the position shown. The examiner prevents
movement of the thigh while applying resistance to the ankle in an inward
direction.

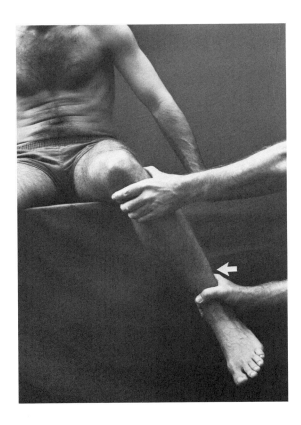

Figure 2-28. External Rotators of the Hip *(obturator externus and internus, gemellus superior and inferior, quadratus femoris, piriformis, gluteus maximus)*

Function: *External (lateral) rotation of the hip.*

Innervation: *Obturator externus: Obturator nerve, L3,* **L4***. Obturator internus: Sacral plexus, L5,* **S1***. Gemellus superior and inferior: Sacral plexus, L5, S1. Quadratus femoris: Obturator nerve, L5, S1. Piriformis: Sacral plexus, L5,* **S1***, S2. Gluteus maximus: Inferior gluteal nerve, L5,* **S1***,* **S2***.*

Comment: *The subject is asked to hold the position shown. The examiner prevents movement of the thigh while applying resistance to the ankle in an outward direction.*

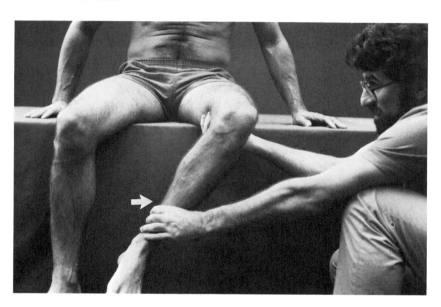

Figure 2-29. Quadriceps Femoris *(rectus femoris, vastus lateralis, vastus medialis, vastus intermedius)*

Function: *Knee extension.*
Innervation: *Femoral nerve, L2,* **L3**, **L4**.
Comment: *The weight of the trunk stabilizes the hip. The examiner supports the subject under his knee to avoid discomfort. Downward resistance is applied at the ankle after the knee has been "locked" into extension. This muscle should not give at all. If the subject cannot complete extension, the grade is less than 3.*

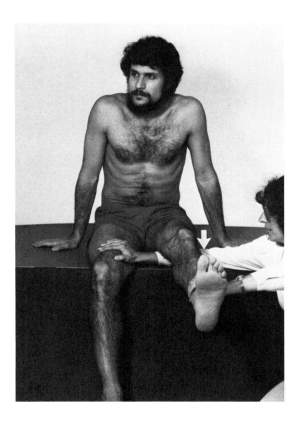

Figure 2-30. Tibialis Anterior

Function: Ankle dorsiflexion and inversion.

Innervation: Deep peroneal nerve, **L4**, L5.

Comment: The subject is asked to dorsiflex and invert her foot (pull it up and in). The examiner applies resistance in a downward and lateral direction. The muscle is very strong and should not give. The tendon can be seen and palpated medially on the dorsum of the ankle.

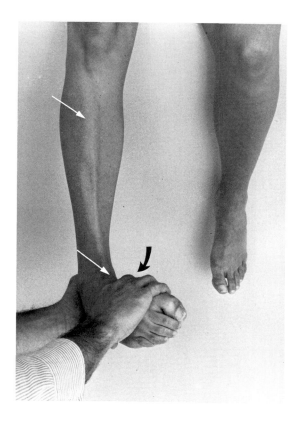

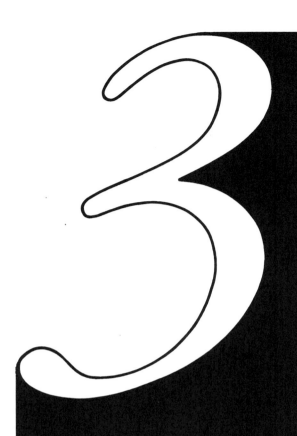

Testing in the
Supine Position

Figure 3-1. Neck Flexors

Function: *Forward flexion of the neck toward the chest.*

Innervation: *Ventral rami of the cervical spinal nerves.*

Comment: *The subject is asked to raise his head off the examining table with his chin tucked in (A). Resistance is applied in a downward and backward direction. The sternocleidomastoids can be tested individually (see Fig. 3-2). (B) Incorrect position for testing the neck flexors. These muscles do not need to contract fully to bring the head to this position, since gravity and the weight of the head will accomplish this. The muscles do contract when resistance is applied, but no grade higher than 4 can be given. If any weakness is shown in this position, the subject must be repositioned and tested in the supine position.*

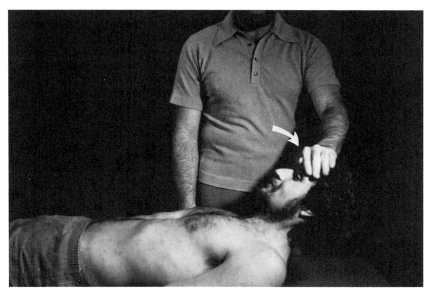

A. Correct

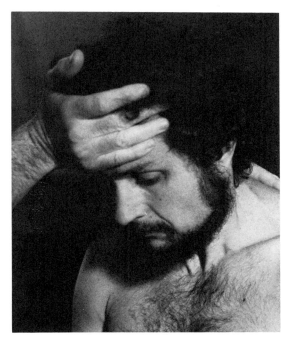

B. Incorrect

Figure 3-2. Sternocleidomastoid

Function: Flexion and lateral rotation of the neck to the opposite side.

Innervation: Accessory nerve (cranial nerve XI).

Comment: In this photograph, the right sternocleidomastoid turns the head to the left. To test it, the examiner applies resistance to the right and downward. The sternocleidomastoid assists the anterior neck flexors.

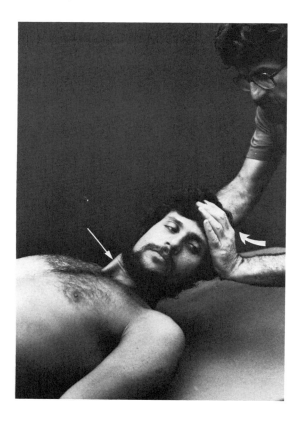

Figure 3-3. Pectoralis Major *(clavicular head)*

Function: Horizontal adduction of the arm.

Innervation: Medial and lateral pectoral nerves, C5 through C8, T1.

Comment: The clavicular portion of the pectoralis major pulls the arm across the chest toward the opposite shoulder. Resistance is given to counteract this movement. This muscle also assists in forward flexion of the arm.

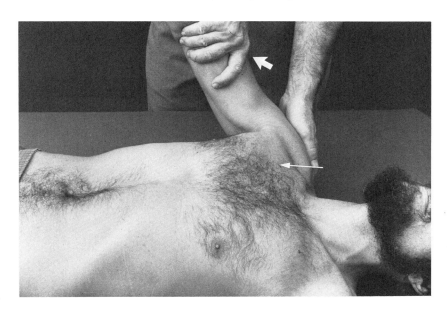

Figure 3-4. Pectoralis Major *(sternal head)*

Function: *Horizontal adduction of the arm.*

Innervation: *Medial and lateral pectoral nerves, C5 through C8, T1.*

Comment: *The subject pulls the arm down and across the chest toward the opposite hip. Resistance is applied (outward and upward) in a direction that counteracts this movement. The examiner is stabilizing the trunk.*

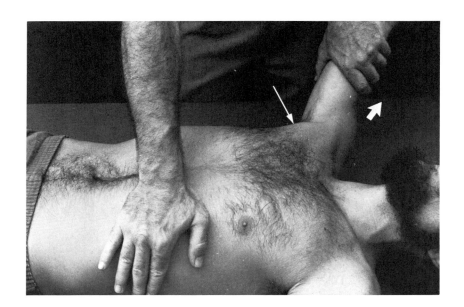

Figure 3-5. Serratus Anterior

Function: *Abduction (protraction) and upward rotation of the scapula.*

Innervation: *Long thoracic nerve, C5, C6, C7.*

Comment: *The subject is asked to reach toward the ceiling with his arm up and slightly abducted (A). Resistance should be applied in a downward direction. The subject's scapula should be lifted completely off the examining table for a grade of 3. For a grade of 5, there should be no scapula movement. In a standing function test of the serratus anterior (B), the subject pushes his extended arm against a wall. With weakness, scapula "winging" may occur. The examiner should watch for movement of the medial border of the scapula away from the thorax.*

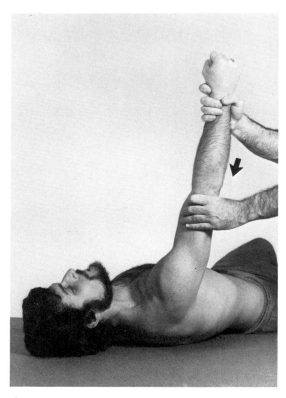

A

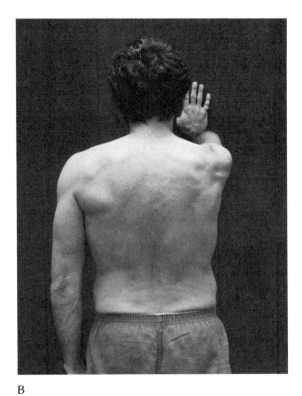

B

Figure 3-6. Abdominals

Function: Flexion of the trunk onto the pelvis anteriorly.

Innervation: T5 through T12.

Comment: The rectus abdominis enables the subject to perform a sit-up. Flexion is assisted by the internal and the external obliques. If the rectus abdominis is weak, the subject may have difficulty raising the head off the table and tilting the pelvis posteriorly. The sit-up should be performed from a supine position on a hard surface with the subject's knees extended. Placement of the hands behind the head makes the test more difficult. It is not necessary for the subject to come up to a full sitting position; he should hold the curled position.

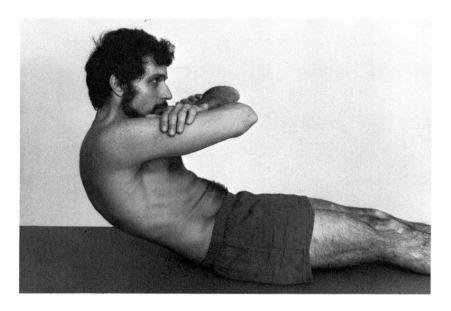

Figure 3-7. Extensor Hallucis Longus

Function: *Extension of the great toe.*

Innervation: *Deep peroneal nerve, L5, S1.*

Comment: *The subject is asked to pull his great toe up and resistance is applied to the base of the great toe in a downward direction. The preferred position is sitting (antigravity). The extensor hallucis longus assists the tibialis anterior in dorsiflexion of the ankle.*

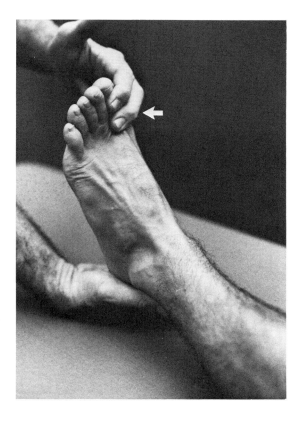

Figure 3-8. Extensor Digitorum Longus and Brevis

Function: *Extension of the toes.*

Innervation: *Deep peroneal nerve, L5, S1, S2.*

Comment: *This photograph demonstrates the combined action of these muscles. The subject is asked to hold his toes up (extended) while the examiner applies resistance in a downward direction. These muscles are not as strong as the extensor hallucis longus. The tendons of the extensor digitorum longus (L) and the belly of the extensor digitorum brevis (B) are easily seen and palpated.*

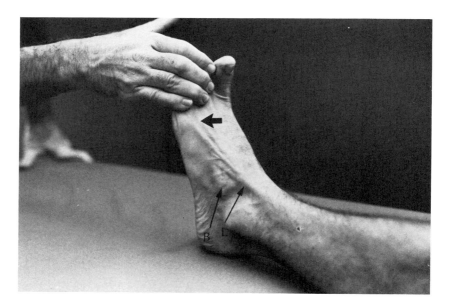

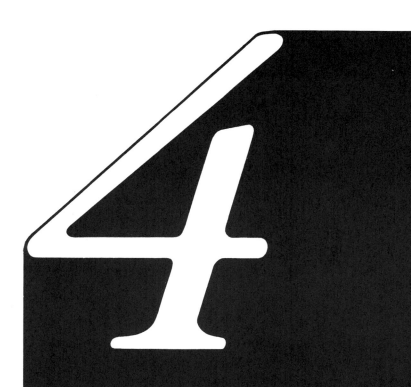

4

Testing in the
Side-lying Position

Figure 4-1. Latissimus Dorsi

Function: *Adduction of the arm and shoulder girdle depression.*

Innervation: *Latissimus dorsi: Thoracodorsal nerve,* **C6**, **C7**, *C8.*

Comment: *This muscle is best tested in the prone position (Fig. 5-7). This photograph (A) shows the muscle belly with the arm positioned at the end of range.*
(B) Incorrect position for testing the latissimus dorsi, since it does not isolate this muscle. The arm is pulled downward by gravity. The pectoralis major and subscapularis are also active.

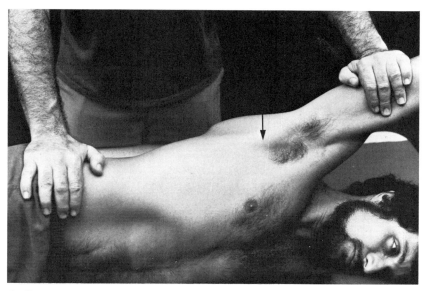

A. Correct

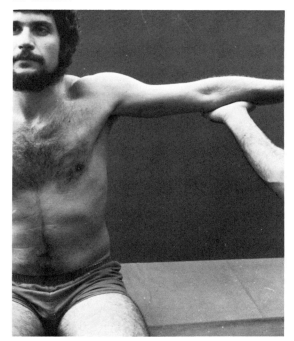

B. Incorrect

Figure 4-2. **Hip Abductors** *(gluteus medius, gluteus minimus, tensor fasciae latae)*

Function: *Hip abduction.*

Innervation: *Gluteus medius, gluteus minimus, superior gluteal nerve,* **L5***, S1. Tensor fasciae latae, superior gluteal nerve, L4, L5.*

Comment: *In the side-lying position (A), the knee and hip should be in extension. The subject may need to hold on to the table for balance. The examiner provides stabilization at the pelvis to avoid trunk rotation. In this incorrect position (B), a weak muscle may escape detection as gravity is eliminated. Even a weak muscle may take resistance and, therefore, cannot be graded properly. The hip abductors should be tested unilaterally.*

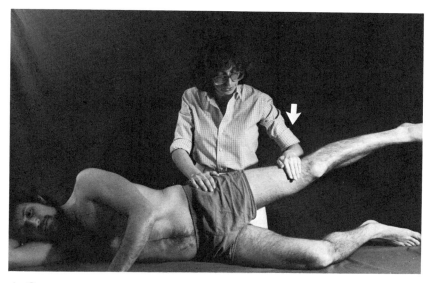

A. Correct

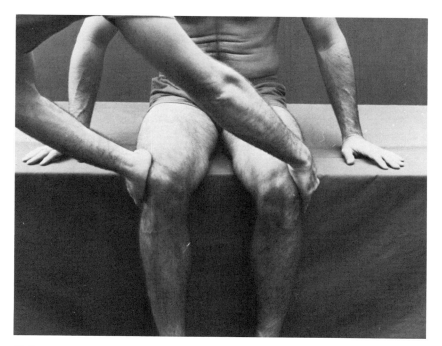

B. Incorrect

Figure 4-3. **Hip Adductors** *(adductor magnus, adductor longus, adductor brevis, gracilis, pectineus)*

Function: *Adduction of the hips.*

Innervation: *Adductor magnus: Obturator and tibial nerves, L2, **L3**, **L4**. Adductor longus and brevis: Obturator nerve, L2, **L3**, L4. Gracilis and pectineus: Obturator nerve, **L2**, L3.*

Comment: *In the side-lying position (A), the upper leg must be fully supported so that the subject is not straining to do both abduction and adduction. The subject is asked to raise the lower leg up while resistance is applied on the lower leg only. These muscles are very strong and should hold in this position. In this incorrect position (B), a weak muscle may escape detection since gravity is eliminated. Even a weak muscle may take some resistance and, therefore, cannot be adequately graded until the subject is repositioned.*

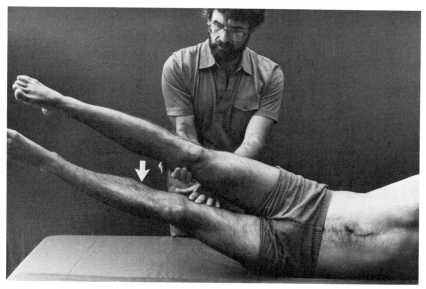

A. Correct

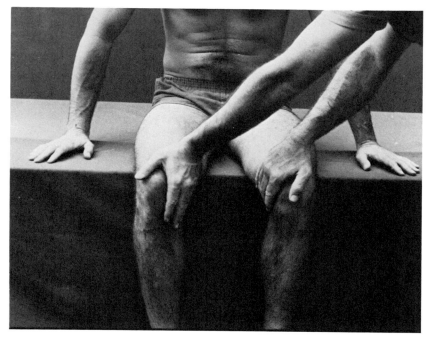

B. Incorrect

Figure 4-4. Peroneus Longus and Brevis

Function: *Eversion of the foot.*
Innervation: *Superficial peroneal nerve,* **L5**, **S1**, *S2.*
Comment: *To test the peroneals, the subject must first plantar flex at the ankle. He should
                   then move the foot outward into eversion. Resistance is applied on the lateral
                   border of the foot in a downward direction toward inversion.*

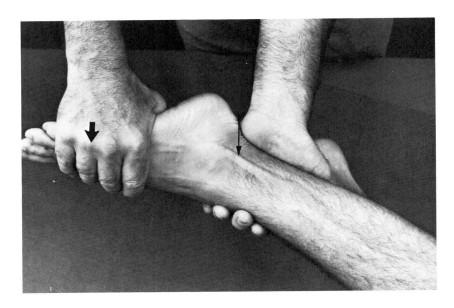

Figure 4-5. Tibialis Posterior

Function: Plantar flexion and inversion.
Innervation: Tibial nerve, L4, L5.
Comment: The examiner stabilizes the ankle and asks the subject to point his foot downward
               and in. Resistance is applied on the instep of the foot in the direction of
               dorsiflexion and eversion.

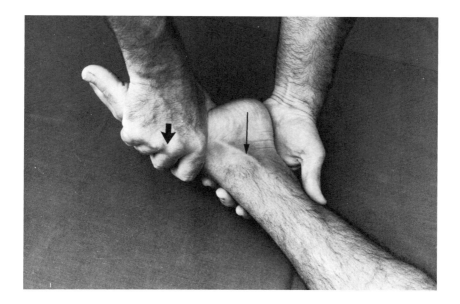

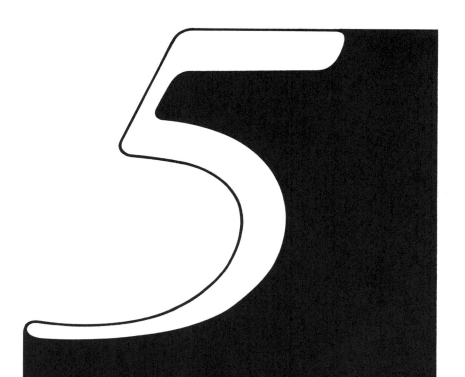

5

Testing in the
Prone Position

Figure 5-1. Neck Extensors

Function: Elevation of the head and extension of the cervical spine.
Innervation: Ventral rami of the cervical spinal nerves.
Comment: In the prone position (A), the superficial and deep paravertebral muscles
                function together. The upper trapezius also assists. (B) Nonstandardized
                (but not incorrect) position for demonstrating function of the posterior neck
                muscle group. The subject must contract these muscles to bring the head
                posteriorly. However, this contraction is assisted by gravity and the weight
                of the head, which can hold the head in this position and can provide the
                feeling of resistance to the examiner. If any weakness is found, the neck extensors
                should be graded in the antigravity position.

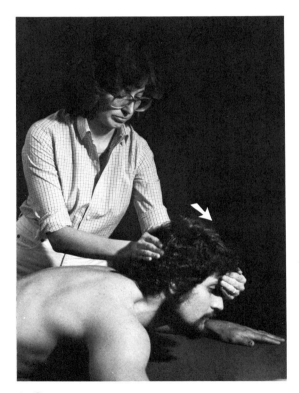

A. Correct

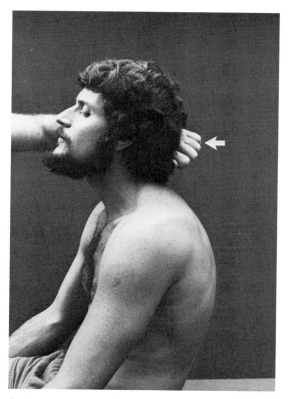

B. Nonstandardized

Figure 5-2. Back Extensors *(erector spinae)*

Function: *Extension of the spine.*

Innervation: *Dorsal rami of the spinal nerves.*

Comment: *This photograph demonstrates a functional test for this group of muscles. The examiner can help stabilize the patient, though the weight of the trunk usually is sufficient.*

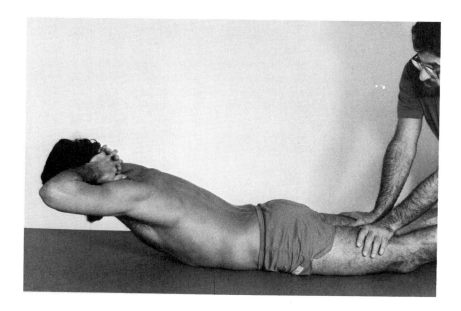

Figure 5-3. Posterior Deltoid

Function: *Horizontal abduction of the shoulder.*

Innervation: *Axillary nerve,* **C5**, *C6.*

Comment: *The subject's arm is positioned over the edge of the table and he is asked to lift his elbow up. The examiner stabilizes the shoulder and scapula. Resistance is given downward and forward toward the edge of the table. Inadequate fixation of the scapula may show spurious posterior deltoid weakness. Alternate position (B) for testing the posterior deltoid, in which the subject pulls the arm backward and upward against the examiner's downward, forward resistance.*

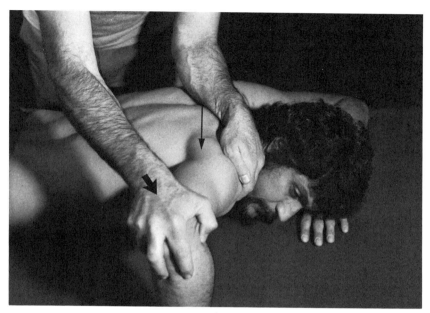

A. Correct

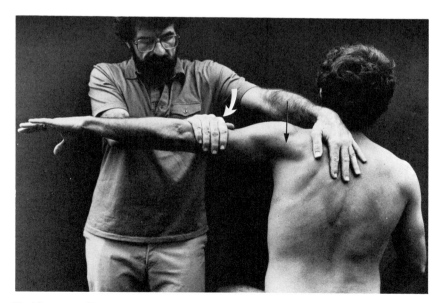

B. Alternate Correct

Figure 5-4. Middle Trapezius

Function: *Adduction of the scapula.*

Innervation: *Accessory nerve (cranial nerve XI).*

Comment: *The subject holds the arm up while the examiner applies resistance to the scapula in a lateral direction. If the posterior deltoid is weak, the examiner must support the arm during testing. For a grade of 5, there should be no scapula abduction.*

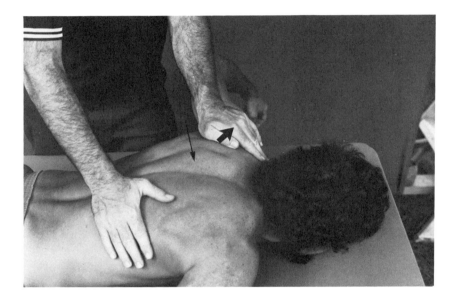

Figure 5-5. Lower Trapezius

Function: Adduction and depression of the scapula.

Innervation: Accessory nerve (cranial nerve XI).

Comment: The subject is positioned with his arm straight and lifted overhead off the examining table. Resistance is applied on the arm in a downward direction. If the deltoid is weak and the patient cannot elevate the arm, the examiner should support the arm and apply resistance against the scapula in the direction of the pull of the lower trapezius.

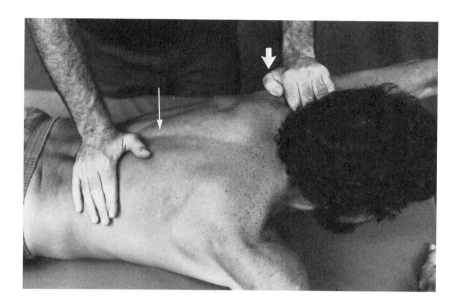

Figure 5-6. Rhomboids

Function: *Adduction and elevation of the scapula.*

Innervation: *Dorsal scapular nerve, upper trunk, C4, C5.*

Comment: *The subject is asked to place his hand near the lower back and lift the elbow up. This movement will adduct the scapula. Resistance can be applied to the scapula in the direction of abduction and upward rotation.*

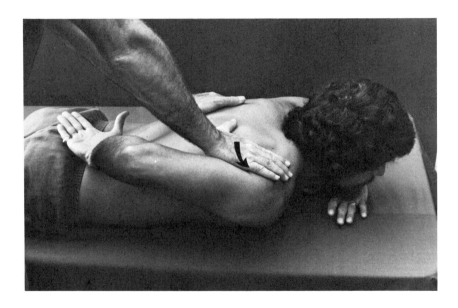

Figure 5-7. Latissimus Dorsi and Teres Major

Function: *Adduction of the arm and shoulder girdle depression.*

Innervation: *Latissimus dorsi, thoracodorsal nerve,* **C6**, **C7**, *C8. Teres major, lower subscapular nerve,* **C6**, *C7.*

Comment: *The subject is asked to adduct and elevate his arm while resistance is applied in an abducted direction. The latissimus dorsi and teres major can be palpated at the inferior angle of the scapula.*

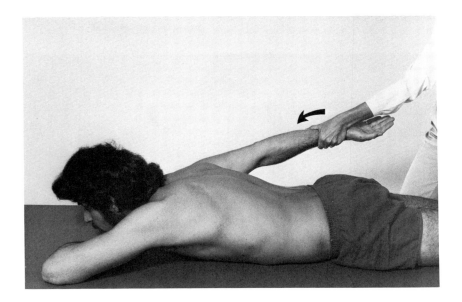

Figure 5-10. Gluteus Maximus

Function: *Hip extension.*

Innervation: *Inferior gluteal nerve, L5,* **S1**, **S2**.

Comment: *Elevation of the thigh to 45 degrees is sufficient (A). If the patient raises the knee much higher, he may rotate his hip and trunk. The examiner stabilizes the opposite hip and applies downward resistance to the lower thigh. The knee must be flexed, or the hamstrings will assist. The gluteus maximus can also be tested in an alternate position (see Fig. 8-17, page 140). In this incorrect position (B), the examiner is pulling up the weight of the limb. Gravity alone pulls the limb down and an accurate strength assessment cannot be made.*

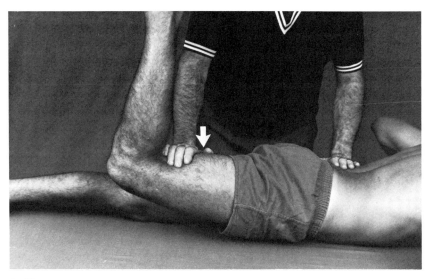

A. Correct

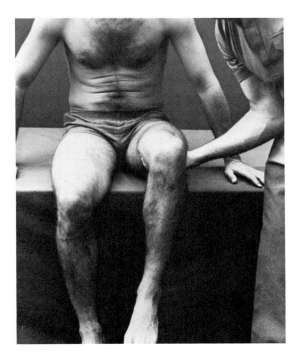

B. Incorrect

Figure 5-11. Hamstrings *(medial: semimembranosus, semitendinosus;*
lateral: biceps femoris)

Function: *Knee flexion.*

Innervation: *Tibial nerve (except the short head of the biceps femoris which is innervated by the peroneal nerve), L5, S1, S2.*

Comment: *The examiner provides stabilization to avoid hip movement (A). To isolate the medial and lateral portions of the hamstrings, resistance can be applied against either of those directions. Subjects may cramp during this test.*
Sitting (B) is an incorrect position for testing the hamstrings, since it is a gravity-assist position. Supine (C) also is an incorrect test position for these muscles.

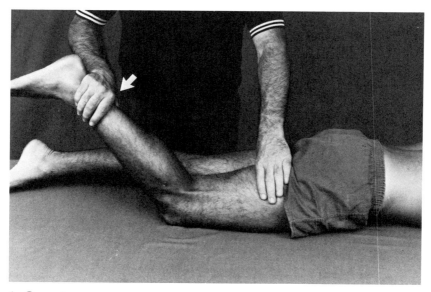

A. Correct

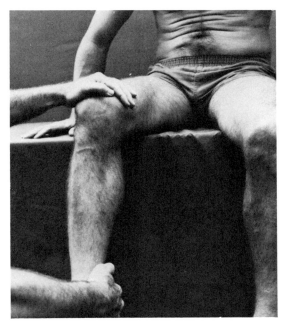

B. Incorrect

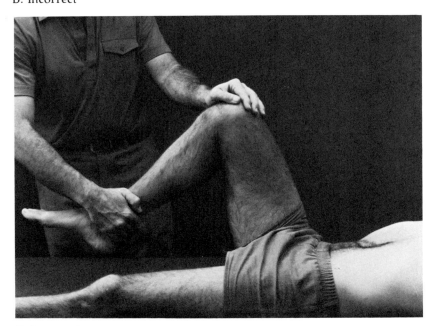

C. Incorrect

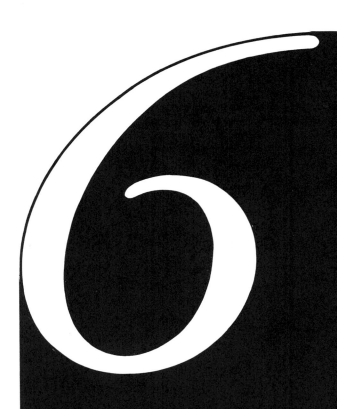

Testing in the
Standing Position

Figure 6-1. Hip Abductors

The Trendelenburg sign as a test for pelvic tilt is useful for assessing the strength of the hip abductors. It complements the isolated test for the gluteus medius in the side-lying position. The pelvic brim should remain horizontal when the subject raises his leg. For a full discussion, see Figure 8-2, page 126.

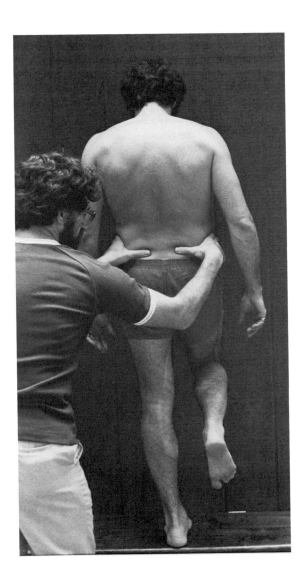

Figure 6-2. Triceps Surae *(gastrocnemius and soleus)*

Function: *Plantar flexion.*

Innervation: *Tibial nerve, S1, S2.*

Comment: *The subject should hold on for balance while lifting the heel off the floor, keeping the knee straight, and the opposite leg raised. A grade of 5 requires that the subject perform this maneuver at least five times. In this incorrect position (B), even weak plantar flexors can withstand a good deal of resistance and, therefore, cannot be adequately tested.*

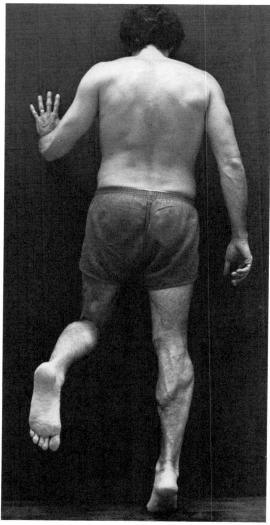

A. Correct

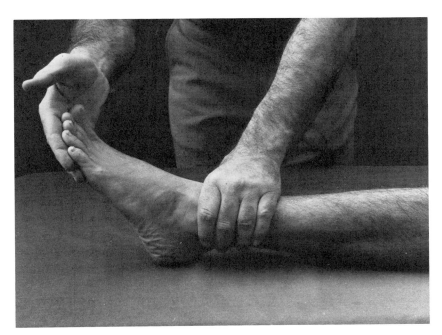

B. Incorrect

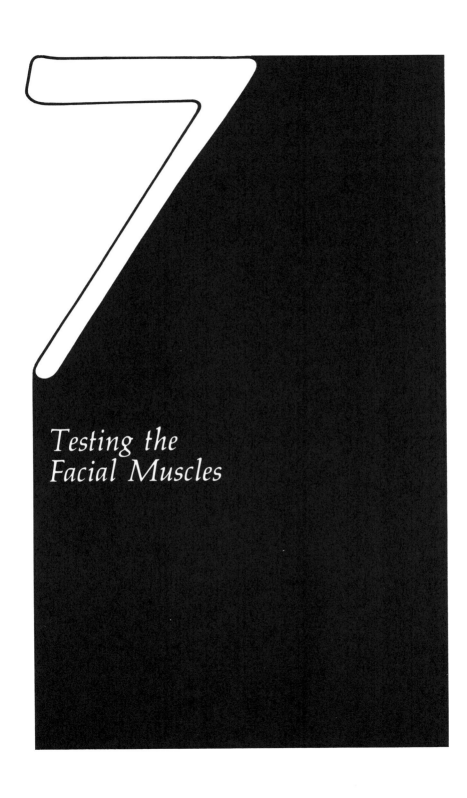

7

Testing the
Facial Muscles

The facial muscles provide movement for expression and are important in chewing and speech. Chewing is the cooperative movement of several muscles. Facial expressions recruit muscles in patterns that vary from individual to individual, although certain lip patterns are stereotyped so that different individuals can produce the same sounds.

All facial muscles are supplied by branches of cranial nerves V (trigeminal) and VII (facial) or from the cervical plexus.

The finer movements of the facial muscles do not lend themselves to manual muscle testing. Observation of the movements and their symmetry is most important. The examiner should demonstrate the movement and have the subject duplicate it. The subject may need a mirror to observe his or her attempts at imitation.

The application of resistance is not often used with facial muscles. However, resistance may be applied to a few muscles (for example, those of jaw opening and closing). Other muscles should be tested by function. It is best to use descriptive terms to designate the amount of active movement (full movement, only initiates movement, and so on). The muscles shown in this chapter are those most frequently tested.

Figure 7-1. Frontalis

Function: *Elevation of the eyebrows.*
Innervation: *Facial nerve.*
Comment: *The subject is asked to raise her eyebrows toward the ceiling without raising her head. The examiner should check for asymmetry of the wrinkles.*

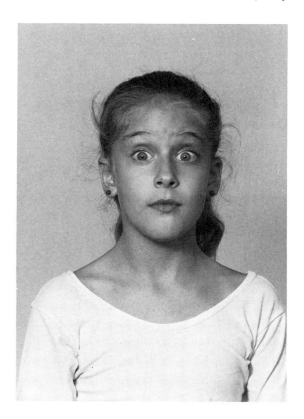

Figure 7-2. Orbicularis Oculi

Function: *Tight eye closure.*

Innervation: *Facial nerve.*

Comment: *Resistance can be applied after the patient squeezes her eyes tightly. The examiner may carefully try to lift the upper eyelid, but if the muscle has full strength, the examiner should not be able to succeed. Passive eyelid closure is accomplished by relaxation of the levator palpebrae superioris. Ptosis is a result of weakness or fatigue of the levator palpebrae superioris, not of the orbicularis oculi.*

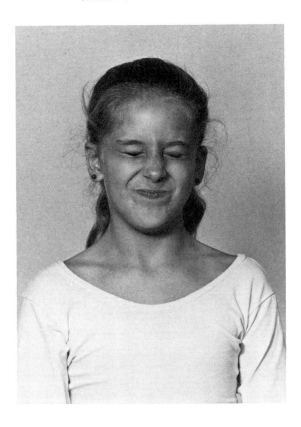

Figure 7-3. Temporalis and Masseter

Function: *Tight jaw closure and chewing.*
Innervation: *Mandibular branch of the trigeminal nerve.*
Comment: *The subject is asked to clench her teeth. Each muscle is palpated indi-*
                 vidually. Resistance can be applied against the chin in a downward direction.
                 The jaw should not open unless the temporalis and masseter are weak. The
                 history should confirm that the patient has difficulty chewing.

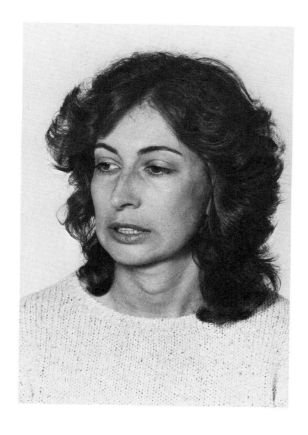

Figure 7-4. Zygomaticus

Function: Turning the corners of the mouth upward (grinning).

Innervation: Facial nerve.

Comment: The patient is asked to show her teeth while smiling. Symmetry of the smile should be observed. Bilateral facial weakness is easily missed, and a transverse smile will result if the zygomaticus is weak.

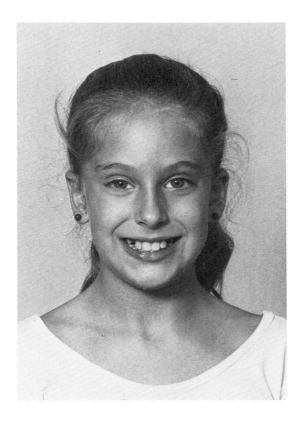

Figure 7-5. Risorius

Function:	Making a straight smile, without upward movement of the corners of the mouth.
Innervation:	Facial nerve.
Comment:	The risorius works with the zygomaticus in smiling.

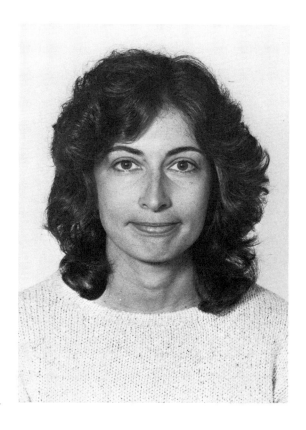

Figure 7-6. Orbicularis Oris

Function: *Compression of the lips as in sucking on a straw; pursing the lips as in whistling.*

Innervation: *Facial nerve.*

Comment: *The subject is asked to perform the functional tests of compressing and pursing the lips.*

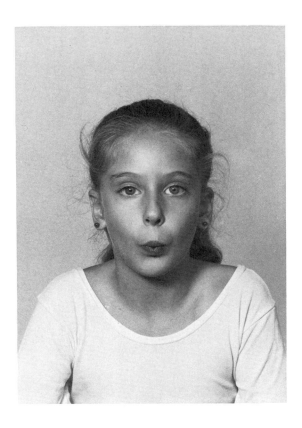

Figure 7-7. **Suprahyoids** *(mylohyoid, geniohyoid, stylohyoid, digastric)*
and Lateral Pterygoids

Function: *Depresses the mandible (opening the jaw) by working together.*
Innervation: *Mixed—facial nerve, trigeminal nerve, and cervical plexus.*
Comment: *The subject is asked to open her mouth. If one of the lateral pterygoids is weak, the jaw will deviate toward the ipsilateral side. Resistance is applied against the jaw in an upward direction. In a normal subject, the jaw should not close.*

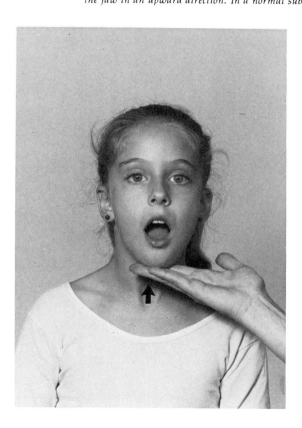

Figure 7-8. Buccinator

Function: *Lines the cheeks; aids in chewing.*
Innervation: *Facial nerve.*
Comment: *The subject often is asked to puff her cheeks with air, a combined function of the buccinator and orbicularis oris. A more isolated action would be blowing as if playing a wind instrument, as shown.*

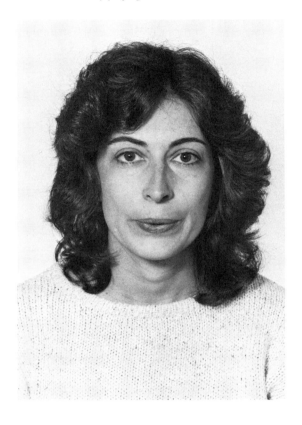

Figure 7-9. Platysma

Function: A superficial muscle that constricts the skin over the anterior neck.
Innervation: Facial nerve.
Comment: The subject is asked to draw the corners of her mouth downward and to tuck
              her chin in. The platysma muscle is not important functionally, but this test
              is useful in checking for symmetry.

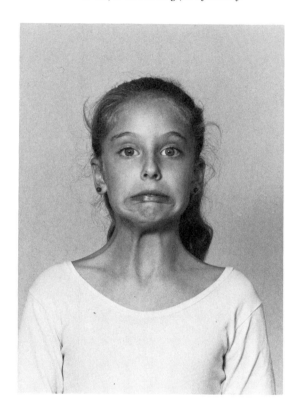

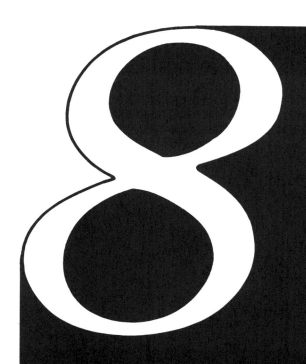

Pediatric Functional
Assessment

Children between the ages of 2 and 5 years may not cooperate in a true manual muscle test. They can initiate a position, but they may not be able to sustain it. They do not understand the counterforce they must exert against the examiner's resistance [12].

The normal child can demonstrate functional ability in everyday play activity. The examiner should be familiar with the performance of children without disabilities and should observe the rhythm, range, and symmetry of their movements during play.

Since children have short attention spans, play may have to be incorporated into functional testing. The positions photographed in this chapter demonstrate normal posture and muscle function. Not every position will work with every child; therefore, some muscles are demonstrated in several positions.

Children's motor abilities mature at different rates [1]. Obese children may have difficulty with some functional tests. Reticence and reluctance to cooperate with the examiner should not be interpreted as weakness.

Isolated muscles are *not* graded in the functional assessment. The muscles or muscle groups observed should be noted as able or unable to perform a function. If the functional test demonstrates weakness in a muscle group, the weakness can be described as mild, moderate, or severe. However, the examiner should realize that these are subjective terms of description.

Before beginning, the child should be undressed down to shorts. The child's posture in sitting or standing should be observed, and the examiner should watch the child walk, run, and jump before more specific tests are attempted.

Figure 8-1. Child Standing
(A) Side view. (B) Posterior view. A mild standing lordosis of the lower back and mild scapula winging are common. The examiner should observe symmetry of the shoulders, hips, leg length, and extremity girth.

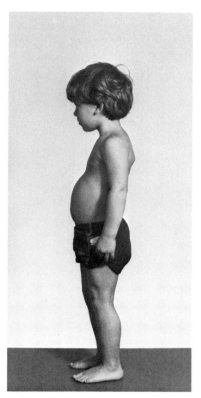 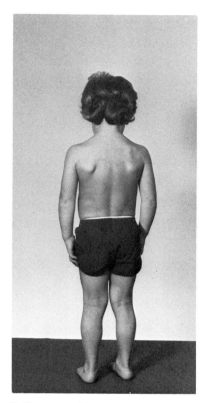

A. Side View   B. Posterior View

Figure 8-2. Test for Lateral Pelvic Tilt

This test demonstrates asymmetry of the hip abductors (gluteus medius and minimus). In the child with normal strength, the pelvis is maintained in horizontal alignment. As the child lifts her left leg, the right hip should remain level. If the pelvis drops on the left side, the right hip abductors are weak. With bilateral hip abductor weakness, the pelvis dips on each side as the child walks, creating a waddling gait.

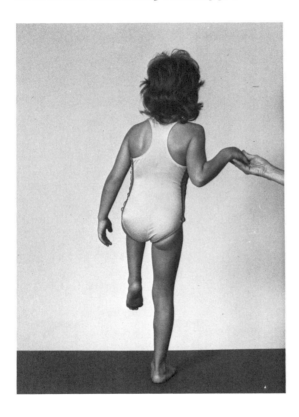

Figure 8-3. Test for Scapular Winging
The child is asked to push his arms forward with palms flat against a wall. The scapula should remain flat against the thoracic wall. A winged scapula may indicate weakness of the serratus anterior.

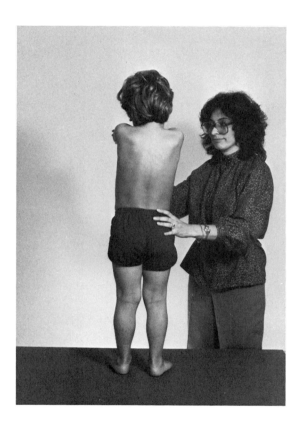

Figure 8-4. Squatting

The ability to rise from a squat demonstrates good strength of the gluteus maximus and quadriceps femoris. The examiner should stand near the child to catch him if he is unsteady.

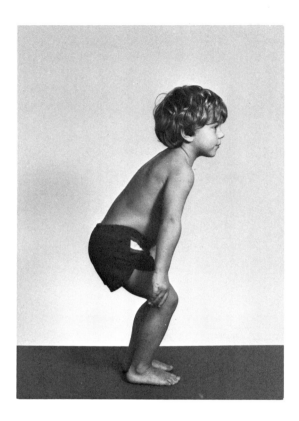

Figure 8-5. Gowers' Maneuver

A child with proximal lower-extremity muscle weakness will climb up her legs using her hands to push off. This indicates hip extensor weakness and her knees may hyperextend. A wide base stance indicates hip weakness.

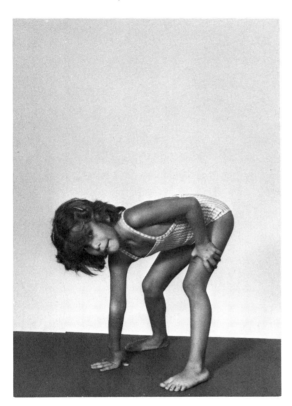

Figure 8-6. Rise from Toe Touching

Performance of this test demonstrates good strength in the back extensors and gluteus maximus.

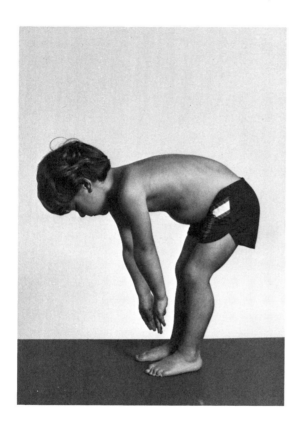

Figure 8-7. Heel Gait

Children older than 3 years should be able to perform this test but may need the assistance of the examiner for balance. As in the adult, this is a functional test of dorsiflexors of the ankle.

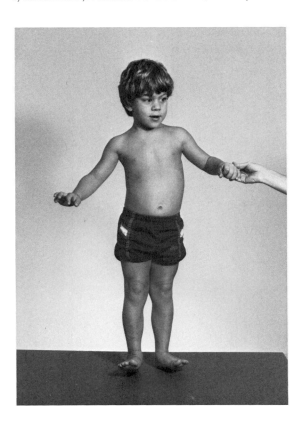

Figure 8-8. Toe Gait

In this test, too, the child may need assistance for balance. Performance of the toe gait demonstrates good strength in the triceps surae (gastrocnemius-soleus group).

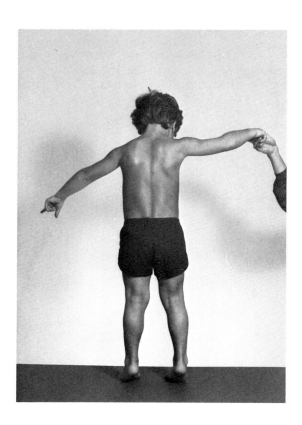

Figure 8-9. Stepping up onto a Stool
The hip flexors and hamstrings raise the leg up onto the stool. The quadriceps femoris and the hip extensors elevate the child.

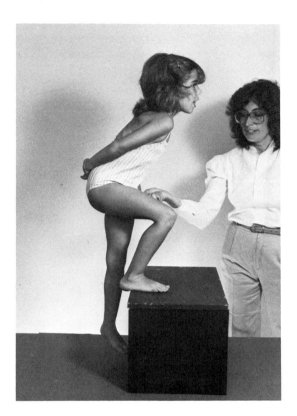

Figure 8-10. Wheelbarrow
The muscles needed to hold this position are the triceps, latissimus dorsi, serratus anterior, and neck extensors.

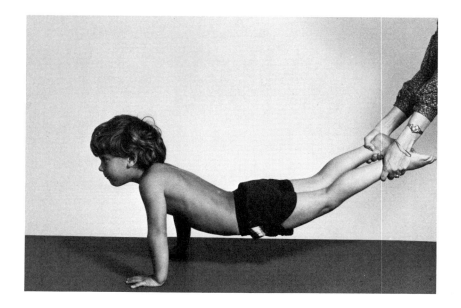

Figure 8-11. Elevation on Hands

This position demonstrates good function of the upper trapezius, latissimus dorsi, scapular depressors (lower trapezius), triceps, and hip flexors. The child may have difficulty with balance and may not be able to hold this position for more than a few seconds. If the child's arms are too short, towels or books may be needed under his hands.

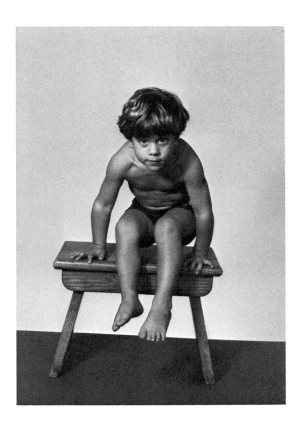

Figure 8-12. Sit-up

A child younger than 6 years has great difficulty doing a sit-up. Abdominal strength is insufficient to lift the trunk off the table or floor. However, an isometric contraction can be palpated. The neck flexors must be strong to initiate the attempted sit-up.

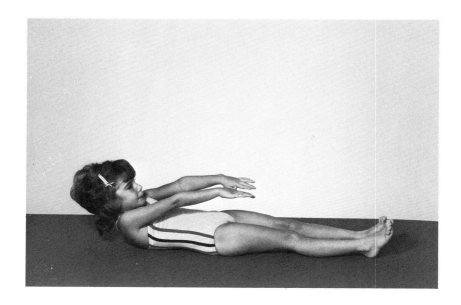

Figure 8-13. Pull to Sitting
If the child is allowed to grasp the examiner's hands and to pull himself to a sitting position, he will use the flexors and intrinsics of the hand and thumb and the biceps. The neck flexors must contract strongly to avoid head lag.

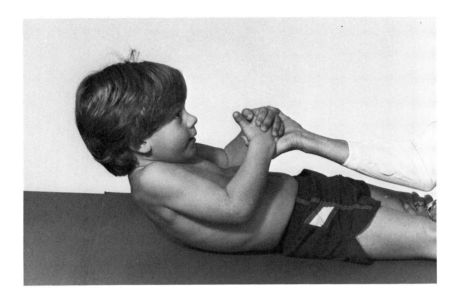

Figure 8-14. Bridging

If the child can perform this test, she demonstrates good strength in the gluteus maximus. The hamstrings maintain the legs in a flexed position. If further height is attempted, she will push down on the balls of her feet using the calf muscles (triceps surae) and toe flexors.

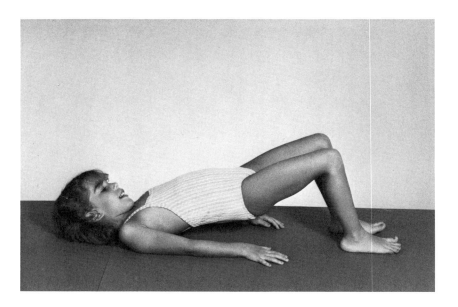

Figure 8-15. Bicycle

The alternating posturing of the legs demonstrates hip and knee flexor strength as the child draws her leg up toward her chest, and hip and knee extensor strength as she lowers it. The examiner should look for control of the legs during the movement.

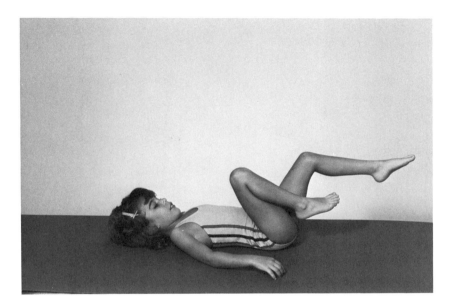

Figure 8-16. Flying
This position is fatiguing, and the child may not be able to sustain it for more than a few seconds. It demonstrates good strength of the back and neck extensors, the middle trapezius, and the posterior deltoid.

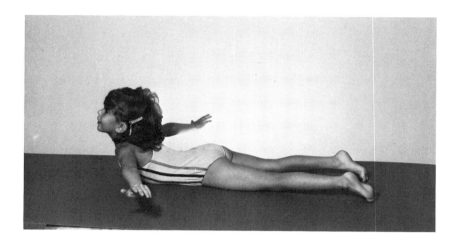

Figure 8-17. Backward Kick *(alternate position for testing the gluteus maximus)*
The child is asked to kick one leg up toward the ceiling. She should keep her knee bent. This enables the gluteus maximus to perform without the assistance of the hamstrings.

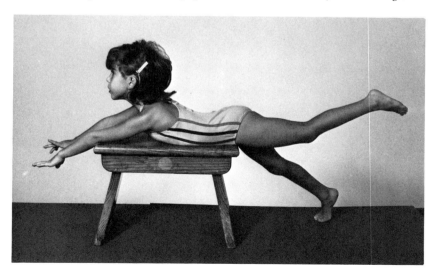

The Denver Developmental Screening Test (DDST) is a standardized screening tool used to recognize developmental and behavioral problems in children aged newborn to 6 years. It is designed for use by paramedical personnel without special training in psychological testing and requires approximately 15 minutes to administer.

There are four testing sections: personal-social, fine motor—adaptive, language, and gross motor skills. A workbook is available which provides a full explanation of how to administer and interpret the test [7]. Items that need further explanation are indicated by a number on the lefthand side of the test item bar. These numbers correspond to footnotes to the test. The letter *R* means that the item can be passed if the parent reports that the child is able to do it. The test requires the examiner to make behavioral observations at the time of testing, noting how the child feels at that time, his or her relation to the tester, the child's attention span, verbal behavior, self-confidence, and so on.

We have included the gross motor skills section of the DDST to serve as a guide to a child's pattern of motor development (Fig. 8-18). The footnotes appropriate to this section are explained in the figure. The interpretation of the gross motor skills section is limited unless all parts of the DDST are administered. As a general rule, if a vertical line is drawn through the patient's age, the child should pass the items to the left of the line. Any items transected by the line need not be passed in normal development. If the child is suspected of having delayed motor development, the full DDST should be administered in conjunction with a full pediatric evaluation.

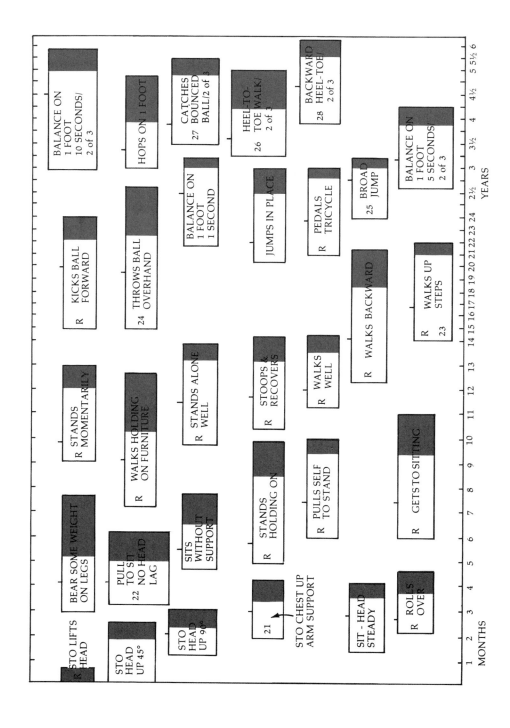

STO = stomach; SIT = sitting.
PERCENT OF CHILDREN PASSING:

25 50 75 90

May pass by report →

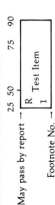

Footnote No. →

21When placed on stomach, child lifts chest off table with support of forearms or hands.
22When child is on back, grasp his or her hands and pull the child to sitting. Pass if the child's head does not hang back.
23Child may use wall or rail only, not person. May not crawl.
24Child must throw ball overhand 3 feet to within arm's reach of tester.
25Child must perform standing broad jump over width of test sheet (8½ inches).
26Tell child to walk forward, ◯◯◯◯ → heel within 1 inch of toe. Tester may demonstrate. Child must walk four consecutive steps, two out of three trials.
27Bounce ball to child who should stand 3 feet away from tester. Child must catch ball with hands, not arms, two out of three trials.
28Tell child to walk backward, ← ◯◯◯◯ toe within 1 inch of heel. Tester may demonstrate. Child must walk four consecutive steps, two out of three trials.

Figure 8-18. Gross Motor Skills Section of the Denver Developmental Screening Test
(*From Frankenburg, Dodds, and Fandal* [7].)

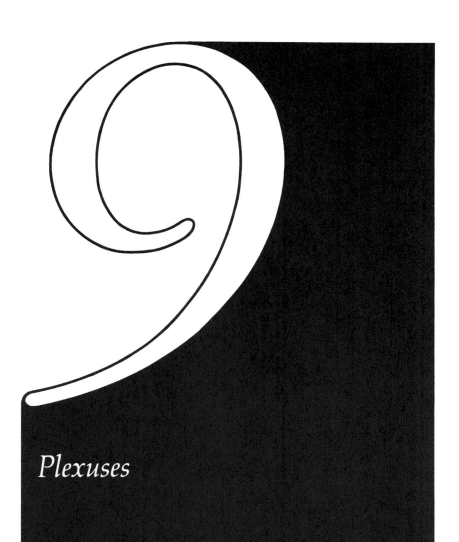

Plexuses

146

Figure 9-1. Brachial Plexus
(Adapted from Kendall, Kendall, and Wadsworth [9]; and J. Patten, Neurological
Differential Diagnosis. *London: Harold Starke Ltd., 1977.)*

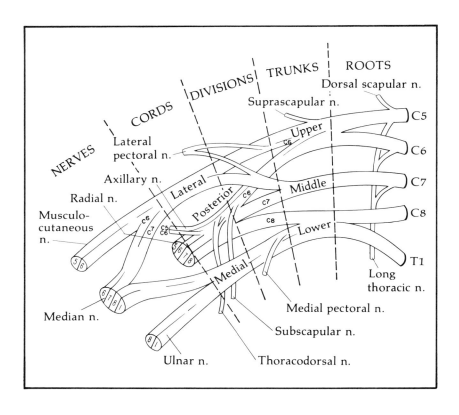

Figure 9-2. Lumbar Plexus

(Adapted from W. Haymaker and B. Woodhall, Peripheral Nerve Injuries *[2nd ed.]. Philadelphia: Saunders, 1953; and R. Warwick and P. L. Williams [Eds.],* Gray's Anatomy *[35th British ed.]. Philadelphia: Saunders, 1973.)*

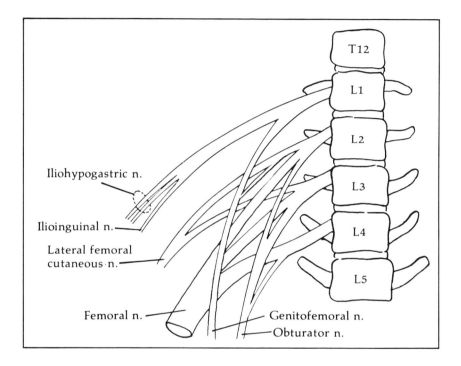

Figure 9-3. Sacral Plexus
(Adapted from R. Warwick and P. L. Williams [Eds.], Gray's Anatomy *[35th British ed.]. Philadelphia: Saunders, 1973.)*

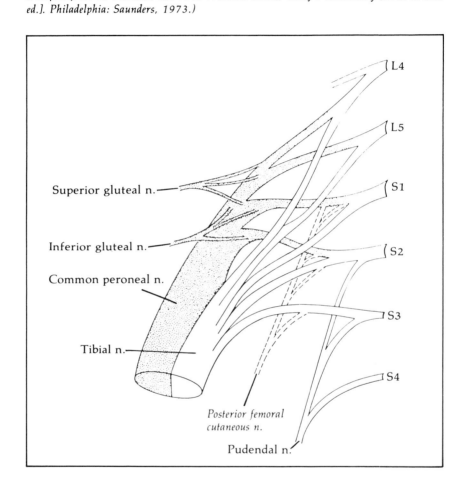

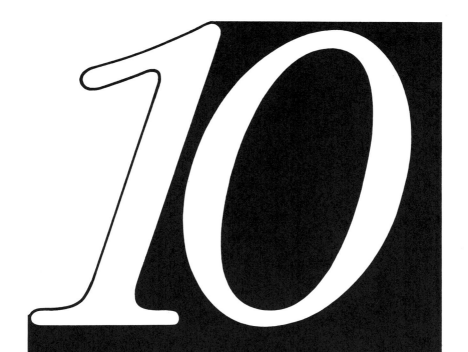

10

Nerves

Figure 10-1. Median Nerve

(A) Median nerve and the muscles supplied by it. (B) Cutaneous branches in the hand (posterior view, left) and cutaneous innervation (anterior view, right) of the median nerve. (Adapted from W. Haymaker and B. Woodhall, Peripheral Nerve Injuries [2nd ed.]. Philadelphia: Saunders, 1953; and the Medical Research Council [11].)

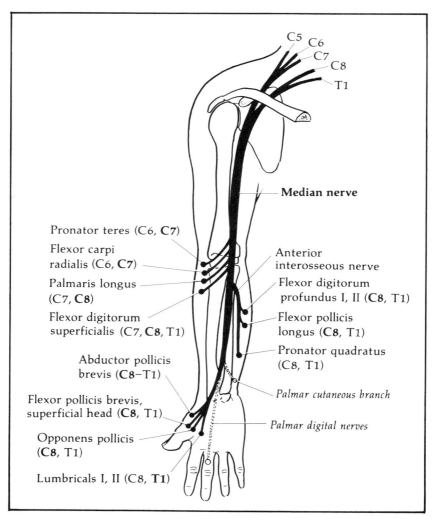

A

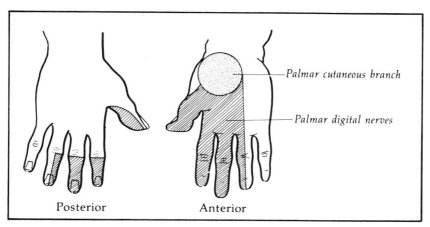

Posterior   Anterior

Palmar cutaneous branch

Palmar digital nerves

B

Figure 10-2. Radial Nerve

(A) Radial nerve and the muscles supplied by it. (B) Patterns of cutaneous innervation, posterior (left) *and anterior* (right) *views. (Adapted from W. Haymaker and B. Woodhall,* Peripheral Nerve Injuries *[2nd ed.]. Philadelphia: Saunders, 1953; and the Medical Research Council [11].)*

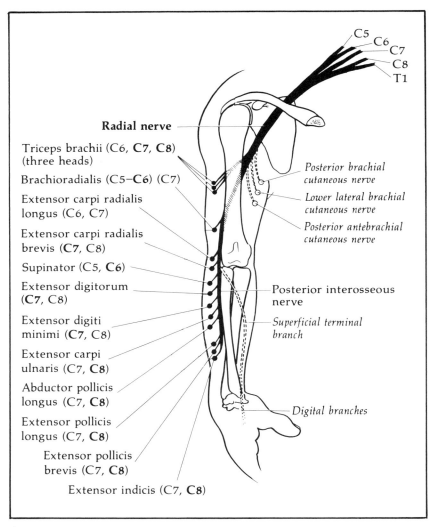

A

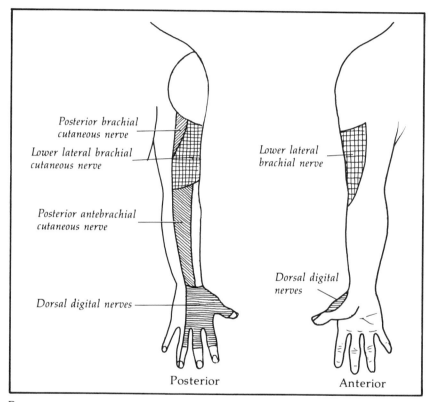

Posterior brachial
cutaneous nerve

Lower lateral brachial
cutaneous nerve

Lower lateral
brachial nerve

Posterior antebrachial
cutaneous nerve

Dorsal digital
nerves

Dorsal digital nerves

Posterior

Anterior

B

Figure 10-3. Ulnar Nerve

(A) Ulnar nerve and the muscles supplied by it. Anterior (left) *and posterior* (right) *views of cutaneous nerve distribution (B) and fields of innervation of the cutaneous branches (C). (Adapted from W. Haymaker and B. Woodhall,* Peripheral Nerve Injuries *[2nd ed.]. Philadelphia: Saunders, 1953; and the Medical Research Council [11].)*

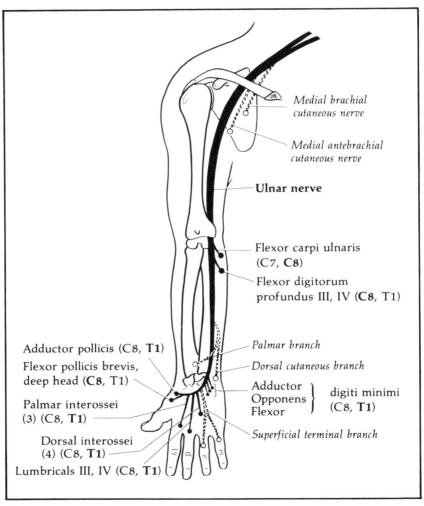

Medial brachial cutaneous nerve

Medial antebrachial cutaneous nerve

Ulnar nerve

Flexor carpi ulnaris (C7, **C8**)

Flexor digitorum profundus III, IV (**C8**, T1)

Adductor pollicis (C8, **T1**)

Flexor pollicis brevis, deep head (**C8**, T1)

Palmar interossei (3) (C8, **T1**)

Dorsal interossei (4) (C8, **T1**)

Lumbricals III, IV (C8, **T1**)

Palmar branch

Dorsal cutaneous branch

Adductor
Opponens } digiti minimi
Flexor (C8, **T1**)

Superficial terminal branch

A

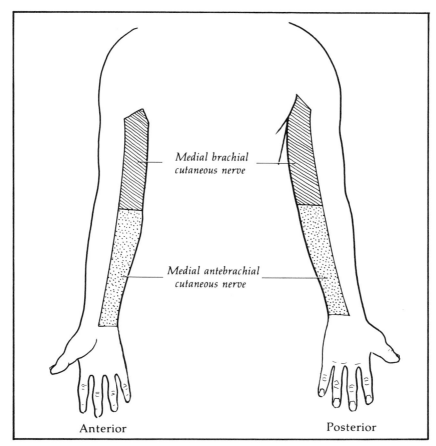

B

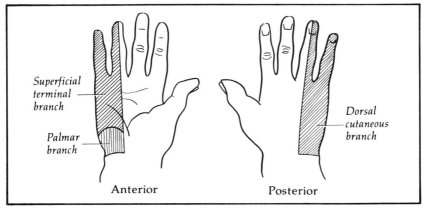

C

Figure 10-4. Femoral Nerve

(A) Femoral nerve and the muscles supplied by it. (B) Cutaneous distribution of the femoral nerve from the anterior (left) *and medial* (right) *aspects. (Adapted from W. Haymaker and B. Woodhall,* Peripheral Nerve Injuries *[2nd ed.]. Philadelphia: Saunders, 1953.)*

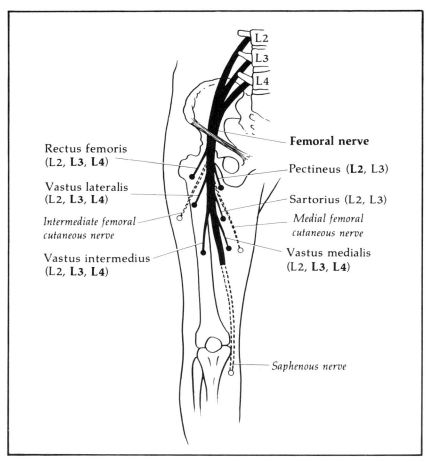

A

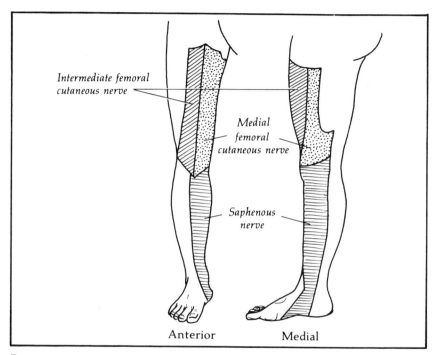

Intermediate femoral
cutaneous nerve

Medial
femoral
cutaneous nerve

Saphenous
nerve

Anterior   Medial

B

158

Figure 10-5. Obturator Nerve

(A) Obturator nerve and the muscles supplied by it. (B) Cutaneous distribution of the obturator nerve from the medial aspect. (Adapted from W. Haymaker and B. Woodhall, Peripheral Nerve Injuries [2nd ed.]. Philadelphia: Saunders, 1953.)

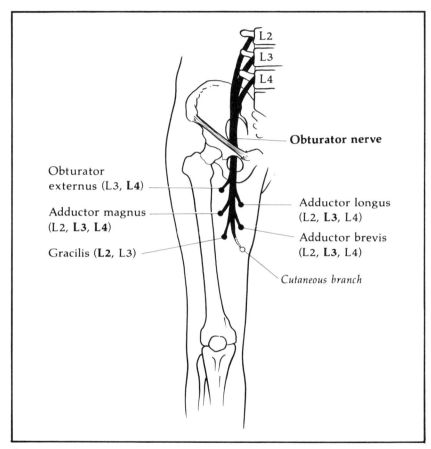

A

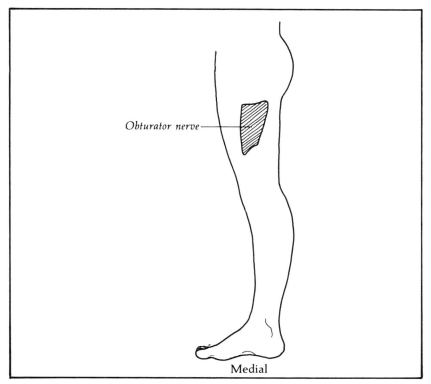

Obturator nerve

Medial

B

Figure 10-6. Sciatic, Tibial, and Plantar Nerves

(A) Sciatic and tibial nerves and the muscles supplied by them. (B) Posterior (left) and medial (right) views of the cutaneous distribution of the sciatic and tibial nerves. (C) Distribution of the plantar nerves. (Adapted from W. Haymaker and B. Woodhall, Peripheral Nerve Injuries *[2nd ed.]. Philadelphia: Saunders, 1953.)*

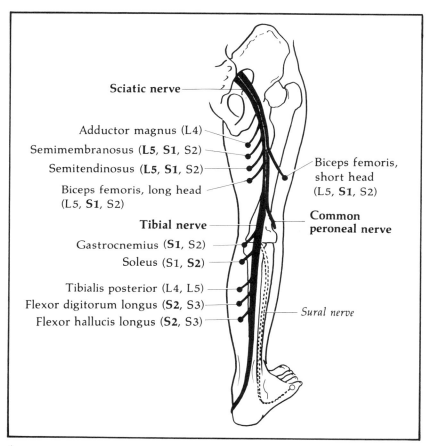

A

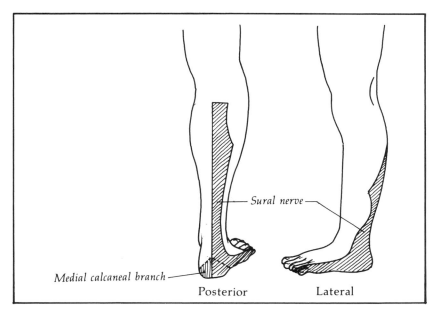

Sural nerve

Medial calcaneal branch

Posterior   Lateral

B

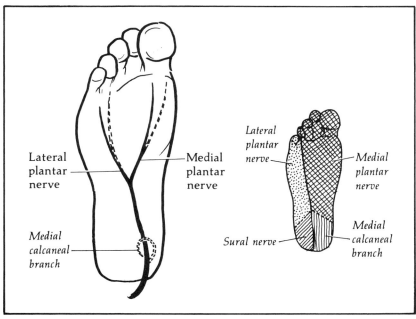

Lateral plantar nerve

Medial plantar nerve

Medial calcaneal branch

Lateral plantar nerve

Medial plantar nerve

Sural nerve

Medial calcaneal branch

C

Figure 10-7. Peroneal Nerve

(A) Peroneal nerve and the muscles supplied by it. (B) Cutaneous distribution of the peroneal nerve. (Adapted from W. Haymaker and B. Woodhall, Peripheral Nerve Injuries *[2nd ed.]. Philadelphia: Saunders, 1953.)*

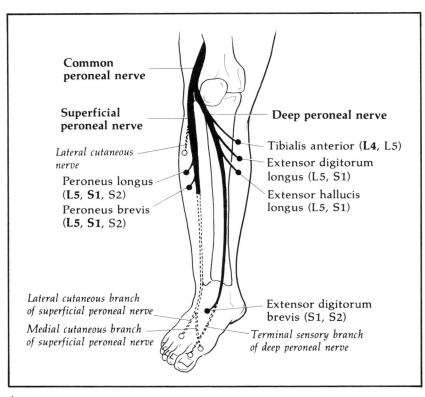

A

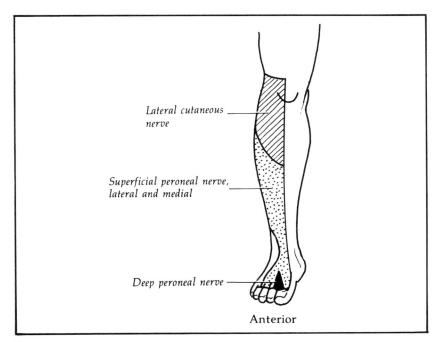

B

11

Dermatomes

Figure 11-1. Dermatomes from the Anterior View

The uppermost dermatome adjoins the cutaneous field of the mandibular division of the trigeminal nerve. The arrows indicate the lateral extensions of dermatome T3. (From W. Haymaker and B. Woodhall, Peripheral Nerve Injuries *[2nd ed.]. Philadelphia: Saunders, 1953. Reprinted by permission.)*

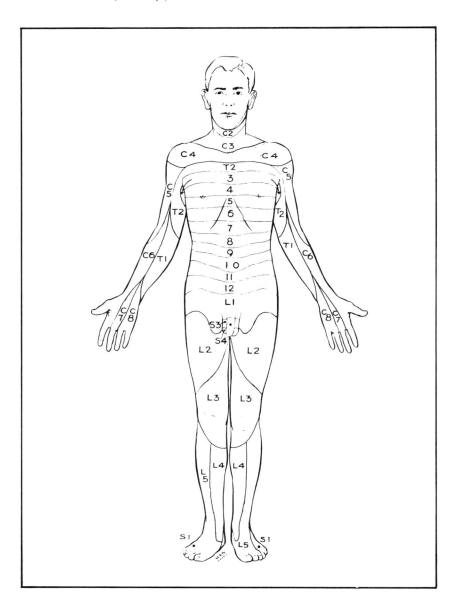

Figure 11-2. Dermatomes from the Posterior View
Note the absence of cutaneous innervation by the first cervical segment. Arrows in the axillary regions indicate the lateral extent of dermatome T3; those in the region of the vertebral column point to the first thoracic, the first lumbar, and the first sacral spinous processes. (From W. Haymaker and B. Woodhall, Peripheral Nerve Injuries *[2nd ed.]. Philadelphia: Saunders, 1953. Reprinted by permission.)*

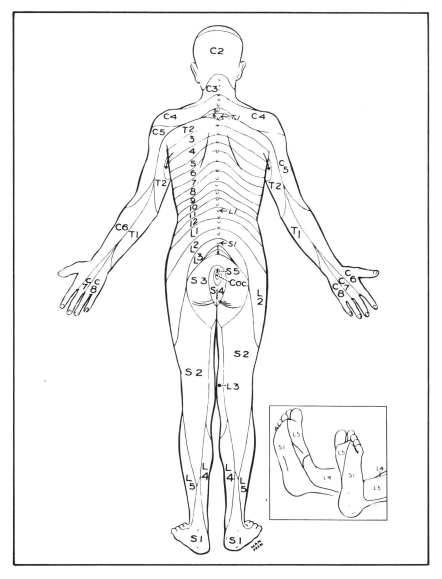

Figure 11-3. Dermatomes from the Side View
(From W. Haymaker and B. Woodhall, Peripheral Nerve Injuries *[2nd ed.].*
Philadelphia: Saunders, 1953. Reprinted by permission.)

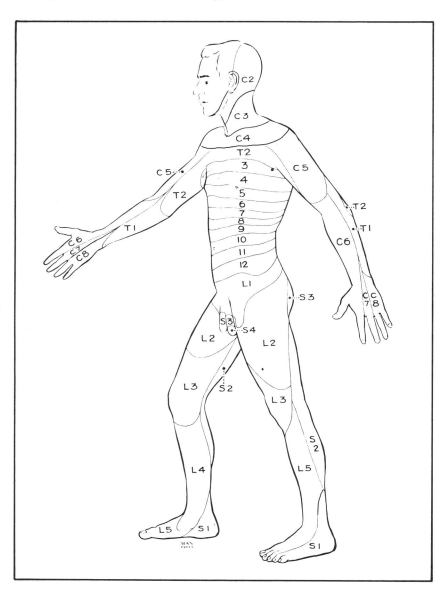

References

1. Alexander, J., and Molnar, G. E. Muscular strength in children: Preliminary report on objective standards. *Arch. Phys. Med. Rehabil.* 54:424, 1973.
2. Basmajian, J. V. *Therapeutic Exercise* (3rd ed.). Baltimore: Williams & Wilkins, 1978.
3. Brunnstrom, S. *Clinical Kinesiology* (3rd ed.). Philadelphia: Davis, 1983.
4. Calliet, R. *Shoulder Pain* (2nd ed.). Philadelphia: Davis, 1981.
5. *Cybex II, Isolated Joint Testing and Exercise: A Handbook for Using Cybex II and the V.B.X.T.* Ronkonkoma, New York: Lumex Inc., 1981.
6. Daniels, L., Williams, M., and Worthingham, C. *Muscle Testing: Techniques of Manual Examination* (4th ed.). Philadelphia: Saunders, 1980.
7. Frankenburg, W. K., Dudds, L. B., and Fandal, A. W. *Denver Developmental Screening Test: Manual and Workbook for Nursing and Paramedical Personnel.* Denver: William K. Frankenburg, 1973.
8. Karpandji, I. A. *The Physiology of the Joints* (5th ed.), Vol. 1. Edinburgh: Livingstone, 1982.
9. Kendall, H. O., Kendall, F. P., and Wadsworth, P. T. *Muscles: Testing and Function* (2nd ed.). Baltimore: Williams & Wilkins, 1971.
10. Lovett, R. W., and Martin, E. G. Certain aspects of infantile paralysis with a descriptive method of muscle testing. *J.A.M.A.* 66:729, 1916.
11. Medical Research Council. *Aids to the Investigation of Peripheral Nerve Injuries* (4th impression). War memorandum, no. 45. London: Her Majesty's Stationery Office, 1982.
12. Molnar, G. E., and Alexander, J. Development of quantitative standards for muscle strength in children. *Arch. Phys. Med. Rehabil.* 55:490, 1974.
13. Murray, M. P., Gardner, G., Mollinger, L., and Sepic, S. Strength of isometric and isokinetic contractions. *Phys. Ther.* 60:412, 1980.
14. Smidt, G. L. Factors contributing to the regulation and clinical assessment of muscle strength. *Phys. Ther.* 62:1283, 1982.

Appendixes

The following appendixes are included to assist the reader in the muscle examination procedure. The forms and tables should simplify the data collection and evaluation as well as provide a logical order in which to conduct the examination. The bibliography (page 186) is a list of recommended readings in the field.

Order of the Examination and Alternate Positions was included to simplify the examination procedure. An alternate position is provided for most muscles.

The Muscle Evaluation Form and the Pediatric Functional Evaluation Form are useful for data collection during the examination of patients. Repeat examinations can be compared, as space for the results of several tests is provided.

The Table of Muscles and Their Innervations is a useful cross reference to the muscle groups described in the text and listed in the two evaluation forms in the Appendix.

Order of the Examination and Alternate Positions

Muscles in preferred testing order and position*	Alternate position for normal subjects*
Sitting	
Facial muscles	Supine
Upper trapezius and levator scapulae	—
Middle and anterior deltoid	—
Triceps brachii	Prone
Biceps brachii and brachioradialis	—
Supinator, pronators	Supine
Wrist and hand flexors and extensors	Supine
Hip flexors	Supine with knee extended
Hip external rotators	—
Hip internal rotators	—
Quadriceps femoris	Supine
Tibialis anterior	Supine
Tibialis posterior	—
Toe extensors	Supine

Supine
    Anterior neck flexors   —
    Sternocleidomastoid   —
    Abdominals   —
    Serratus anterior   Sitting or standing
    Pectoralis major   Sitting for clavicular head

Side-lying
    Gluteus medius   Lateral pelvic tilt in standing
                                position
    Hip adductors   —
    Peroneals   Sitting
    Latissimus dorsi   Prone

Prone
    Neck extensors   Sitting
    Back extensors   —
    Triceps brachii   Sitting
    Posterior deltoid   Sitting
    Middle trapezius   —
    Rhomboids   Sitting
    Latissimus dorsi   Side-lying
    Gluteus maximus   Standing
    Hamstrings   Standing

Standing
    Gastrocnemius-soleus   —

---

*Subjects with weakness may need to be tested in gravity-eliminated positions. See Daniels et al. in the Bibliography.

Muscle Evaluation Form

Patient's name: _____

Chart #: _____

Date of birth: _____

Handedness: _____

Grading scale

0	No contraction	0%
1	Trace	20%
2	Poor	40%
3	Fair	60%
4	Good	80%
5	Normal	100%

	Right					Left		
				Date/Examiner				
				Face				
				Frontalis				
				Orbicularis oculi				
				Buccinator/orbicularis oris				
				Risorius/zygomaticus				
				Masseter/temporalis				
				Neck				
				Flexors				
				Sternocleidomastoid				
				Extensors				
				Scapula				
				Upper trapezius				
				Serratus anterior				
				Middle trapezius				
				Lower trapezius				
				Rhomboids				

				Shoulder				
				Anterior deltoid				
				Middle deltoid				
				Posterior deltoid				
				Pectoralis major				
				Latissimus dorsi and teres major				
				Internal rotators				
				External rotators				
				Upper extremity				
				Triceps brachii				
				Biceps brachii				
				Brachioradialis				
				Supinator				
				Pronators				
				Wrist extensors R/U				
				Wrist flexors R/U				
				Extensor digitorum				
				Flexor digitorum superficialis				
				Flexor digitorum profundus				
				Dorsal interossei				
				Lumbricals				
				Palmar interossei				
				Thumb				
				Flexor pollicis longus/brevis				
				Extensor pollicis longus/brevis				
				Adductor pollicis				
				Abductor pollicis longus/brevis				
				Opponens pollicis				

				Hip				
				Iliopsoas				
				Gluteus maximus				
				Gluteus medius and minimus				
				Adductors				
				Lower extremity				
				Quadriceps femoris				
				Hamstrings				
				Tibialis anterior				
				Tibialis posterior				
				Peroneals longus/brevis				
				Gastrocnemius-soleus				
				Toe extensors				
				Toe flexors				
				Extensor hallucis				
				Flexor hallucis				
				Trunk				
				Upper abdominals				
				Lower abdominals				
				Lateral abdominals				
				Internal obliques				
				External obliques				
				Back extensors				

Descriptive data:

Gait:

Posture:

Trendelenburg Sign (Lateral Pelvic Tilt):

Scoliosis:

Gowers' maneuver:

Areas of pain (spasticity):

Pediatric Functional Evaluation Form

Patient's name: ⎯⎯⎯⎯⎯⎯⎯⎯⎯⎯

Date of birth: ⎯⎯⎯⎯⎯⎯⎯⎯⎯⎯

Diagnosis: ⎯⎯⎯⎯⎯⎯⎯⎯⎯⎯

Handedness: ⎯⎯⎯⎯⎯⎯⎯⎯⎯⎯

Grading key

N	Normal
M	Mild difficulty
Mo	Moderate difficulty
S	Severe difficulty

Right		Functional Activity	Muscles Involved	**Left**	
		Date/Examiner			
		Lateral Pelvic Tilt— Trendelenburg sign	Gluteus medius		
		Push arms forward	Serratus anterior		
		Rise from squat	Gluteus maximus		
			Quadriceps femoris		
		Rise from toe touching	Back extensors		
			Gluteus maximus		
		Heel gait	Tibialis anterior		
			Extensor hallucis longus		
		Toe gait	Gastrocnemius-soleus		
		Stepping up onto stool	Hip flexors		
			Hamstrings		
			Quadriceps femoris		
			Hip extensors		
		Wheelbarrow	Triceps brachii		
			Latissimus dorsi		
			Serratus anterior		

		Elevation on hands	Upper trapezius		
			Triceps brachii		
			Latissimus dorsi		
			Lower trapezius		
			Serratus anterior		
		Sit-up	Neck flexors		
			Rectus abdominis		
		Pull to sitting	Biceps brachii		
			Finger flexors		
			Intrinsics of hand		
			Wrist flexors		
			Neck flexors		
		Bridging	Gluteus maximus		
		Bicycle	Hip flexors		
			Quadriceps femoris		
		Flying	Neck extensors		
			Back extensors		
		Backward kick	Gluteus maximus		

Descriptive data:

Posture:

Gait:

Running, jumping:

Denver Developmental Scale:

Table of Muscles and Their Innervation

Muscle(s)	Innervation
Abdominals	*See* Obliquus externus abdominis, obliquus internus abdominis, rectus abdominis
Abductor digiti minimi	Ulnar nerve, C8, **T1**
Abductor pollicis brevis	Median nerve, **C8**, T1
Abductor pollicis longus	Posterior interosseous nerve (from radial nerve), C7, **C8**
Adductor brevis	Obturator nerve, L2, **L3**, L4
Adductor longus	Obturator nerve, L2, **L3**, L4
Adductor magnus	Obturator and tibial nerves, L2, **L3, L4**
Adductor pollicis	Ulnar nerve, C8, **T1**
Back extensor Erector spinae	Dorsal rami of spinal nerves
Biceps brachii	Musculocutaneous nerve, lateral cord, C5, **C6**
Biceps femoris, long head	Tibial nerve, L5, **S1**, S2
Biceps femoris, short head	Peroneal nerve, L5, **S1**, S2
Brachialis	Musculocutaneous nerve, lateral cord, C5, **C6**, radial nerve, (C7) to small lateral part of muscle
Brachioradialis	Radial nerve, C5, **C6**, (C7)
Buccinator	Facial nerve
Coracobrachialis	Musculocutaneous nerve, lateral cord, C5, **C6**, C7
Deltoid (anterior, middle, posterior fibers)	Axillary nerve, posterior cord, **C5**, C6
Diaphragm	Phrenic nerve, C3, **C4**, C5
Digastric	*See* Suprahyoids
Erector spinae	*See* Back extensor
Extensor carpi radialis brevis	Posterior interosseous nerve (from radial nerve), **C7**, C8
Extensor carpi radialis longus	Radial nerve, C6, C7
Extensor carpi ulnaris	Posterior interosseous nerve (from radial nerve), C7, **C8**
Extensor digiti minimi	Posterior interosseous nerve (from radial nerve), **C7**, C8

Muscle(s)	Innervation
Extensor digitorum	Posterior interosseous nerve (from radial nerve), **C7**, **C8**
Extensor digitorum brevis	Deep peroneal nerve, S1, S2
Extensor digitorum longus	Deep peroneal nerve, L5, S1
Extensor hallucis brevis	Deep peroneal nerve, L5, S1
Extensor hallucis longus	Deep peroneal nerve, L5, S1
Extensor indicis	Posterior interosseous nerve (from radial nerve), C7, **C8**
Extensor pollicis brevis	Posterior interosseous nerve (from radial nerve), C7, **C8**
Extensor pollicis longus	Posterior interosseous nerve (from radial nerve), C7, **C8**
Finger extensors	*See* Extensor digiti minimi, extensor digitorum, extensor indicis
Finger flexors	*See* Flexor digiti minimi, flexor digitorum profundus, flexor digitorum superficialis
Flexor carpi radialis	Median nerve, C6, **C7**
Flexor carpi ulnaris	Ulnar nerve, C7, **C8**
Flexor digiti minimi brevis	Ulnar nerve, C8, **T1**
Flexor digitorum brevis	Medial plantar nerve (from tibial nerve), S2, **S3**
Flexor digitorum longus	Tibial nerve, **S2**, S3
Flexor digitorum profundus I, II	Anterior interosseous branch of median nerve, **C8**, T1
Flexor digitorum profundus III, IV	Ulnar nerve, **C8**, T1
Flexor digitorum superficialis	Median nerve, C7, **C8**, T1
Flexor hallucis brevis	Medial plantar nerve (from tibial nerve), S2, **S3**
Flexor hallucis longus	Tibial nerve, **S2**, S3
Flexor pollicis brevis, deep head	Ulnar nerve, **C8**, T1
Flexor pollicis brevis, superficial head	Median nerve, **C8**, T1
Flexor pollicis longus	Anterior interosseous branch of median nerve, **C8**, T1
Frontalis	Facial nerve
Gastrocnemius	Tibial nerve, **S1**, S2
Gemellus inferior	Sacral plexus, L5, S1
Gemellus superior	Sacral plexus, L5, S1
Geniohyoid	*See* Suprahyoids
Gluteus maximus	Inferior gluteal nerve, L5, **S1**, **S2**

Muscle(s)	Innervation
Gluteus medius	Superior gluteal nerve, **L5**, S1
Gluteus minimus	Superior gluteal nerve, **L5**, S1
Gracilis	Obturator nerve, **L2**, L3
Hamstrings	*See* Biceps femoris, semimembranosus, semitendinosus
Hip abductors	*See* Gluteus medius, gluteus minimus, tensor fasciae latae
Hip adductors	*See* Adductor brevis, adductor longus, adductor magnus, gracilis, pectineus
Hip extensors	*See* Gluteus maximus
Hip external rotators	*See* Gemellus superior and inferior, obturator externus and internus, piriformis, quadratus femoris
Hip flexors	*See* Iliacus, psoas major, tensor fasciae latae
Hip internal rotators	*See* Gluteus medius, gluteus minimus
Iliacus	Femoral nerve, **L2**, L3
Iliopsoas	*See* Iliacus, and psoas major
Infrahyoidei	
Sternohyoid	Ansa cervicalis
Sternothyroid	Ansa cervicalis
Omohyoid	Ansa cervicalis
Thyrohyoid	Branch from hypoglossal nerve and fibers from first cervical spinal nerve
Infraspinatus	Suprascapular nerve, (C4), **C5**, C6
Intrinsics of hand	*See* Dorsal interossei, lumbricals, palmar interossei
Interossei, dorsal	Ulnar nerve, C8, **T1**
Interossei, palmar	Ulnar nerve, C8, **T1**
Knee extensors	*See* Quadriceps femoris
Knee flexors	*See* Gracilis, hamstrings, popliteus
Latissimus dorsi	Thoracodorsal nerve, posterior cord, **C6**, **C7**, C8
Levator scapulae	Spinal nerves C3, C4, dorsal scapular nerve
Lumbricals I, II	Median nerve, C8, **T1**
Lumbricals III, IV	Ulnar nerve, C8, **T1**

Muscle(s)	Innervation
Masseter	Mandibular branch of trigeminal nerve
Mylohyoid	*See* Suprahyoids
Neck extensors	Ventral rami of cervical spinal nerves
Neck flexors	Ventral rami of cervical spinal nerves. *Also see* Sternocleidomastoid
Obliquus externus abdominis	Ventral rami of T6–T12
Obliquus internus abdominis	Ventral rami of T7–L1
Obturator externus	Obturator nerve, L3, **L4**
Obturator internus	Sacral plexus, L5, **S1**
Opponens digiti minimi	Ulnar nerve, C8, **T1**
Opponens pollicis	Median nerve, **C8**, T1; sometimes a twig from deep terminal branch of ulnar nerve
Orbicularis oculi	Facial nerve
Orbicularis oris	Facial nerve
Palmaris longus	Median nerve, C7, C8
Pectineus	Obturator nerve, **L2**, L3
Pectoralis major (clavicular and sternal fibers)	Medial and lateral anterior pectoral nerves, C5, C6, C7, C8, T1
Pectoralis minor	Medial and lateral anterior pectoral nerves, C6, **C7**, C8
Peroneus brevis	Superficial peroneal nerve, **L5**, **S1**, S2
Peroneus longus	Superficial peroneal nerve, **L5**, **S1**, S2
Piriformis	Sacral plexus, L5, **S1**, S2
Platysma	Cervical branch of facial nerve
Popliteus	Tibial nerve, L4, L5, S1
Pronator quadratus	Anterior interosseous branch of median nerve, C8, T1
Pronator teres	Median nerve, C6, **C7**
Psoas major	Ventral rami of lumbar nerves, **L1**, **L2**, L3
Pterygoid, lateral	Anterior trunk of mandibular nerve
Quadratus femoris	Obturator nerve, L5, S1

Muscle(s)	Innervation
Quadratus lumborum	Ventral rami of twelfth thoracic and upper three or four lumbar nerves
Quadriceps femoris (rectus femoris, vastus intermedius, vastus lateralis, vastus medialis	Femoral nerve, L2, **L3**, **L4**
Rectus abdominis	Ventral rami of T5–T12
Rectus femoris	*See* Quadriceps femoris
Rhomboids	Dorsal scapular nerve, upper trunk, C4, **C5**
Risorius	Facial nerve
Sartorius	Femoral nerve, L2, L3
Scapular abductors	*See* Serratus anterior
Scapular adductors	*See* Rhomboids, trapezius
Scapular depressors	*See* Lower trapezius, serratus anterior
Scapular elevators	*See* Levator scapulae, rhomboids, serratus anterior, upper trapezius
Semimembranosus	Tibial nerve, **L5**, **S1**, S2
Semitendinosus	Tibial nerve, **L5**, **S1**, S2
Serratus anterior	Long thoracic nerve, C5, **C6**, **C7**
Shoulder abductors	*See* Biceps brachii, deltoid, supraspinatus
Shoulder adductors	*See* Latissimus dorsi, pectoralis major, teres major, triceps (longhead)
Shoulder extensors	*See* Latissimus dorsi, posterior deltoid, teres major, triceps (longhead)
Shoulder external rotators	*See* Infraspinatus, posterior deltoid, teres minor
Shoulder flexors	*See* Anterior deltoid, biceps femoris, pectoralis major, (coracobrachialis)
Shoulder internal rotators	*See* Latissimus dorsi, pectoralis major, subscapularis, teres major
Soleus	Tibial nerve, S1, **S2**
Sternocleidomastoid	Accessory nerve (cranial nerve XI); branches from C2, C3, ventral rami are mostly sensory

Muscle(s)	Innervation
Stylohyoid	*See* Suprahyoids
Subscapularis	Upper and lower subscapular nerves, posterior cord, C5, **C6**, (C7)
Supinator	Posterior interosseous nerve (from radial nerve), C5, **C6**
Suprahyoids	
Digastric	Anterior belly: Inferior alveolar nerve (from mandibular branch of trigeminal nerve)
	Posterior belly: Facial nerve
Geniohyoid	First cervical spinal nerve through hypoglossal nerve
Mylohyoid	Inferior alveolar nerve (from mandibular branch of trigeminal nerve)
Stylohyoid	Facial nerve
Supraspinatus	Suprascapular nerve, upper trunk, C4, **C5**, C6
Temporalis	Mandibular branch of trigeminal nerve
Tensor fasciae latae	Superior gluteal nerve, L4, L5
Teres major	Lower subscapular nerve, posterior cord, **C6**, C7
Teres minor	Axillary nerve, posterior cord, (C4), **C5**, C6
Tibialis anterior	Deep peroneal nerve, **L4**, L5
Tibialis posterior	Tibial nerve, L4, L5
Toe extensors	*See* Extensor digitorum longus and brevis, extensor hallucis longus and brevis
Toe flexors	*See* Flexor hallucis longus and brevis, flexor digitorum longus and brevis
Trapezius	Accessory nerve (cranial nerve XI), sensory fibers from C3, C4
Triceps brachii	Radial nerve, posterior cord, C6, **C7**, **C8**
Triceps surae	*See* Gastrocnemius, soleus
Vastus intermedius, lateralis, and medialis	*See* Quadriceps femoris

Muscle(s)	Innervation
Wrist extensors	*See* Extensor carpi radialis, extensor carpi ulnaris
Wrist flexors	*See* Flexor carpi radialis, flexor carpi ulnaris
Zygomaticus	Facial nerve

Bibliography

Alexander, J., and Molnar, G. E.   Muscular strength in children: Preliminary report on objective standards. *Arch. Phys. Med. Rehabil.* 54:424, 1973.

Basmajian, J. V.   *Therapeutic Exercise* (3rd ed.). Baltimore: Williams & Wilkins, 1978.

Basmajian, J. V.   *Muscles Alive: Their Function Revealed by Electromyography* (4th ed.). Baltimore: Williams & Wilkins, 1978.

Brunnstrom, S.   *Clinical Kinesiology* (3rd ed.). Philadelphia: Davis, 1983.

Calliet, R.   *Shoulder Pain* (2nd ed.). Philadelphia: Davis, 1981.

Daniels, L., Williams, M., and Worthingham, C.   *Muscle Testing: Techniques of Manual Examination* (4th ed.). Philadelphia: Saunders, 1980.

Falkel, L.   Plantar flexor strength testing using the Cybex isokinetic dynamometer. *Phys. Ther.* 58:847, 1978.

Frankenburg, W. K., Dudds, L. B., and Fandal, A. W.   *Denver Developmental Screening Test: Manual and Workbook for Nursing and Paramedical Personnel.* Denver: William K. Frankenburg, 1973.

Haymaker, W., and Woodhall, B.   *Peripheral Nerve Injuries* (2nd ed.). Philadelphia: Saunders, 1953.

Karpandji, I. A.   *The Physiology of the Joints* (5th ed.), Vols. 1–3. Edinburgh: Livingstone, 1982.

Kendall, F. P., and McCreary, E. K.   *Muscles: Testing and Function* (3rd ed.). Baltimore: Williams & Wilkins, 1983.

Legg, A. T.   The early treatment of poliomyelitis and the importance of physical therapy. *J.A.M.A.* 107:633, 1936.

Licht, S. (Ed.).   *Therapeutic Exercise* (2nd ed.). Baltimore: Elizabeth Licht, 1965. Pp. 163–256.

Lovett, R. W.   *The Treatment of Infantile Paralysis* (2nd ed.). Philadelphia: P. Blakiston, 1917.

Lovett, R. W., and Martin, E. G.   Certain aspects of infantile paralysis with a descriptive method of muscle testing. *J.A.M.A.* 66:729, 1916.

Medical Research Council.   *Aids to the Investigation of Peripheral Nerve Injuries.* War memorandum, no. 45. London: Her Majesty's Stationery Office, 1982.

Molnar, G. E., and Alexander, J. Development of quantitative standards for muscle strength in children. *Arch. Phys. Med. Rehabil.* 55:490, 1974.

Murray, M. P., Gardner, G., Mollinger, L., and Sepic, S. Strength of isometric and isokinetic contractions. *Phys. Ther.* 60:412, 1980.

Patten, J. *Neurological Differential Diagnosis.* London: Harold Starke, 1977.

Smidt, G. L. Factors contributing to the regulation and clinical assessment of muscle strength. *Phys. Ther.* 62:1283, 1982.

Warwick, R., and Williams, P. L. (Eds.). *Gray's Anatomy* (35th British ed.). Philadelphia: Saunders, 1973.

Wright, W. G. *Muscle Function.* New York: Hoeber, 1928.

Index